Never
Never
NEVER
Give up

*An Inspiring
MS Journey*

*blessings on you
Joy Neufeld*

M. Joy (Willms) Neufeld

BALBOA
PRESS
A DIVISION OF HAY HOUSE

ISBN: 978-1-4525-4936-1 (sc)
ISBN: 978-1-4525-4935-4 (e)
ISBN: 978-1-4525-4934-7 (hc)

Library of Congress Control Number: 2012907955

Balboa Press books may be ordered through booksellers or by contacting:

Balboa Press
A Division of Hay House
1663 Liberty Drive
Bloomington, IN 47403
www.balboapress.com
1-(877) 407-4847

Because of the dynamic nature of the Internet, any web addresses or links contained in this book may have changed since publication and may no longer be valid. The views expressed in this work are solely those of the author and do not necessarily reflect the views of the publisher, and the publisher hereby disclaims any responsibility for them.

The author of this book does not dispense medical advice or prescribe the use of any technique as a form of treatment for physical, emotional, or medical problems without the advice of a physician, either directly or indirectly. The intent of the author is only to offer information of a general nature to help you in your quest for emotional and spiritual well-being. In the event you use any of the information in this book for yourself, which is your constitutional right, the author and the publisher assume no responsibility for your actions.

Any people depicted in stock imagery provided by Thinkstock are models, and such images are being used for illustrative purposes only. Certain stock imagery © Thinkstock.

Printed in the United States of America

Balboa Press rev. date: 07/23/2012

A N O V E L BASED ON A TRUE STORY

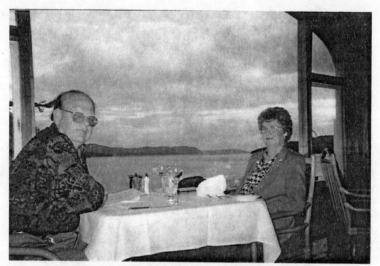

Franz and Heidi dining in an elegant restaurant at Orcas Island.

CONTENTS

PROLOGUE

This is Heidi's long health journey. It began when she was four years old. Due to losing her mother to a debilitating disease and subsequently death, her life became very challenging. Heidi attained tenacity through her mother's loving and embracing influence when she was only four years old.

She was sixteen when a sports injury left her partially paralyzed.

Due to her mother's untimely death, Heidi did not have the nurturing she desperately needed. Because of much anger in the home, Heidi grew up severely wounded.

Heidi married at a young age and soon thereafter Heidi suffered with inflammation in her body due to infections. Dose after dose of antibiotics were prescribed, all to no avail. Was this damaging to her immune system?

This was followed with debilitating fatigue, plus stiff legs which hampered her walking ability.

Heidi worked very hard to find an answer to her dilemma and she found one, because she will NEVER GIVE UP.

Follow her journey in this inspiring book!

GRATITUDE

An attitude of gratitude wells up within me. My husband Don has been there for me on this hazardous windy road. You hold my hand and walk with me all along my journey. You truly meant it when we spoke our wedding vows, "In sickness and in health, till death do us part." Thank you

To our children, Denise, Steven and Lisa. For the years of inconsistencies you put up with in my parenting due to debilitating fatigue and mood swings. Love, kindness, and patience describe you, my beautiful family. You've also put up with not so popular menu ideas that I gave you for your health. I could go on. THANKYOU from the bottom of my heart with all my love.

To Denise and her husband George, to Steve and his wife Sheila and to Lisa and her husband Doug, THANKYOU for taking up the challenge of trying to live healthy lives. THANKYOU for teaching our grandchildren to eat healthy. I love your comments about remembering from your childhood how important it was to eat your vegetables and stay away from eating too much sugar, candy and ice cream. Thank you for observing in your children the foods their bodies do not tolerate well, and for helping them to understand that. Bless you for that!

Thank you to my myriad of friends who have been there for me. The support I felt from you has been full of love and understanding. Thank you for embracing me, time and time again. Thank you for listening, I appreciate you!

Editor   Zachary Schroeder

Thank you so much for the wonderful work you have done for me in editing my book. I so appreciate your time and attention to the wording, which is extraordinaire! You are a very gifted writer.

SOARING   HIGHER

DIGGING   DEEPER

GOING   FURTHUR

WHO COULD HAVE IMAGINED

Never Never NEVER Give Up

AN INSPIRING MS JOURNEY

CHAPTER ONE

FRANZ AND HEIDI

A beautiful sunny day dawned. It was Canada Day, July 1st. The birds chirped loudly waking Heidi from a deep slumber.

"Oh Franz, is it that time already?" asked Heidi as she yawned and rubbed her eyes.

"I'm afraid it is Heidi," responded Franz as he snapped the last button on his blue plaid shirt. "It's time to go for my walk," Franz smiled as he pecked Heidi's cheek. "See you at supper." Franz shut the bedroom door so Heidi could get some more sleep.

"Oh, my legs," Heidi complained as she sat up at the edge of the bed.

"Why do they feel so stiff and heavy?" she wondered. "I sure wish someone had a few answers for me. Oh well, I guess that's my lot in life." murmured Heidi as she pushed herself to her feet. "One day, maybe I'll get some answers." Heidi had her breakfast and swept the kitchen floor. "That's all I've done this morning and I'm already very tired. I have to sit down," Heidi thought to herself.

Heidi sat down on the beige brocade couch in the family room. She turned the television on and noticed black spots in her line of vision. As she looked at the T.V. Heidi noticed two of everything.

"What is going on?" she questioned. "Why am I seeing double? I guess this is another weird action my body is having. I'll have a good night's sleep and it will probably go away."

Heidi had learned over the years that her body wasn't normal like other people's seemed to be. She, however did not have pain, so was very grateful for that.

Walking was a problem and at times she fell! "Why do I trip over my own feet?" Heidi questioned. On a good day Heidi and Franz went for a walk. When Heidi got tired her right leg behaved weirdly. It would bend out of shape, almost twisting. Heidi would have to sit down on the curb while Franz walked home to get the car. Heidi could not walk any further.

At the end of the day Franz came home to dinner. "How was your day?" greeted Franz warmly.

"It has been interesting," replied Heidi. "This morning when I looked at the T.V., I noticed two black spots in my line of vision. As I continued to watch T.V. my eyes saw double of everything."

Franz hugged Heidi. He knew she struggled with her body.

"If it continues tomorrow, I'll go see an optometrist," sighed Heidi.

That evening, Franz and Heidi went to see some friends.

"While we were travelling on the road, I noticed the centre yellow lines were double. I saw two yellow lines crossing each other," said Heidi. "The blacktop too, looked like two roads crossing each other in front of me. But I have no pain or weird feelings in my head. It will disappear," thought Heidi.

The next morning, there were no changes in her eyesight. She would have to go see the optometrist. He would tell her what was wrong.

Heidi made an appointment for that afternoon. She drove to her appointment, parked the red convertible, and sat down in the office. Heidi was quickly ushered into the optometrist's office where he had a look at her eyes. He was startled!

"This is not something I can help you with. You must go to the hospital," he insisted.

Heidi was shocked! She left the office, stepped into her car and drove home.

Franz got home from work and Heidi spoke, "The optometrist insists I go to the hospital. I don't know what this is all about. I guess in time we'll find out."

Franz and Heidi soon entered the hospital. After some time the doctor spoke, "What is the problem?"

"I am seeing double and we were told to come here and see the doctor," spoke Heidi.

The doctor soon checked her eyes. Then he called two more doctors as he didn't have an answer. The other doctors were puzzled as well.

Finally, one spoke, "go see an opthamologist on Monday."

"Yes, we will," sighed Heidi.

The following Monday morning, Franz took Heidi to the eye specialist. He was a very kind, gentle doctor.

He took his instruments and peered into Heidi's eyes. "Do you have numbness in your face?" he questioned. "Have you lost taste in your tongue?"

"No problems there," Heidi replied.

He continued, "If you did, I would suggest you've either had a stroke or you have Multiple Sclerosis. Don't even think of any of those possibilities. You've probably got a virus. It will last for six weeks and then disappear."

The following day, Heidi sat on the couch and wondered, "Am I going to be blind? Why is my eyesight affected?"

"More questions," thought Heidi. " Will they ever end?"

CHAPTER 2

OUR CHERISHED MOTHER

The air was charged with excitement! "We are going on a picnic, we are going on a picnic!" The children chorused.

What a family! This family of two boys and six girls were a lively bunch. They were a fun- loving family who loved to picnic together. Heidi, the middle child, danced around in the large kitchen. She clapped her little hands excitedly.

It was a gorgeous, sunny day. Mom and the girls quickly prepared a delicious lunch. There was fried chicken, potato salad. There were carrot and celery sticks, hot buttered rolls, and a delicious chocolate cake. Everything was placed into the picnic basket. Now they were ready to roll!

Dad picked up the basket and set it into the car. "Get your shoes on Heidi. We're going to leave without you if you don't hurry up," called Dad.

"I'll hurry, " spoke Heidi as her blond pigtails bobbed. She quickly ran back into the house. Poor Heidi. She had been so excited to go on this picnic, she had run outside without her shoes.

"Okay, let's go," announced Dad loudly.

The children piled into the car chatting away. Down the gravel country road they drove with rocks and dust flying.

"Don't sit so close to me," complained Dorrie, "You're squishing me."

"I am not," retorted Elly.

"You are so."

"You kids get along back there, or we'll go home," demanded Dad. They knew they'd better settle down or else.

They drove an hour into the country and found a beautiful park. There was a creek running through it. Tall evergreen trees provided shade for their picnic table. They found the perfect spot. After dad parked the car, he took the picnic basket out of the trunk while the kids scrambled out of the car. Heidi ran off and climbed up the slide. Whish, down she slid.

"Come on, Heidi, don't you want lunch first? Aren't you hungry?" called Mother.

Hurriedly, Heidi came running and sat down at the table. "That slide is so much fun," panted Heidi, all out of breath.

Dad taught this family to say grace before they ate the delicious food. "Thank you Jesus for this food, Amen!" chorused the children.

Then everyone dug in. They were so busy eating there was little chatting happening. Suddenly, one by one they noticed Mother. She'd fallen against Dad with her head down.

Dad laid his roll onto the table and spoke, "Children, your mother is not feeling well. " Dad sat there for a few minutes trying to help their mother. Finally, he announced quietly, "We must go home."

The family had so much love for their mother. One by one they came over and spoke, "I love you so-o-o-o much," as they hugged her.

They looked at their Dad. "We will have to go back home," Dad spoke softly. The sweet children knew something was horrifically wrong. This was a short picnic, but mother needed help.

While Dad gently picked up their loving mother, the kids watched with fear and terror! The mood was very somber. Henry, the older brother, ran to the car and opened the door so Dad could place their mother on the seat. Mother leaned against the seat with her head back and eyes closed.

"I can't move," Mother whispered.

The children slowly sat down to finish their meal. No one was very hungry now. "What is happening to our mother?" all the children thought to themselves.

When Dad finished settling their mother on the front seat of the car, he returned to the table. "I have to take your mother to the hospital, she is very sick. Let's finish eating. You girls can then clear the table. Put everything into the basket and we will drive back home."

Soon the family were on their way. It was a very quiet ride home. Their tears were on the surface. None of the children lamented over the seats in the back anymore. They all focused on their dear mother. These children knew they were each loved and cherished by their mother.

"Now what?" they thought as each one felt a lone tear trickle down their cheek.

Poor Papa. He looked extremely worried. He kept glancing at his dear wife. The children watched as he'd reach out to take her hand and gently squeeze it. They loved each other dearly.

Heidi's mind was frantic! Such a young innocent four year old was worried about the loss of one of the most important people in her life? "This isn't fair," thought Heidi. She could hardly stand to see her mother go through this pain! Heidi wanted it all to stop and be normal. "What is going to happen?" she cried.

Soon Papa was on his way to the hospital. He knew the children would get into bed. Little did he know what lay ahead.

He said, "God, what is going on here? My wife is very sick!"

When he got to the hospital, he gently carried his wife through the doors of the hospital and lay her on a bed.

The doctor came over and asked, "What is happening here?"

Dad took his hat off and spoke, "Our family was having a picnic when my wife collapsed. She cannot move her arms and legs."

The doctor questioned, "When did this happen?"

"A few hours ago," Dad responded quietly.

The doctor picked up his instruments and carefully and methodically tested and checked her body.

After a half hour, the kind doctor spoke, "We do not have any answers for you now. We will admit her and do a lot more testing in the following days. I am sorry I don't have more answers for you," spoke the doctor gently.

Dad kissed his wife and spoke, "I'll be back tomorrow. Maybe they'll have more answers by then."

Dad hated to leave his wife alone but he knew she was very ill and that was the best place for her. He slowly walked away from her bed and blew a kiss as he waved goodbye.

As he walked out of the hospital door, his mind was in a fog. "What could be happening to my wife?" he agonized.

Back home, "What could happen to Mama?" asked Heidi, as Dorrie, the eldest sister put her to bed. "I don't know," sighed Dorrie, "But I hope she gets better soon. We need her."

"Yes, we do," spoke Heidi. "My little finger hurts and Mommy is not here to kiss it."

Dorrie quickly kissed her little finger and said, "You go to sleep now. Goodnight." As the eldest of the girls, Dorrie felt responsible.

Little did anyone guess how long this separation from mother and family would be. One could not imagine what this poor mother was going through. As she lay in that hospital bed week after week, she so longed to be at home with her family.

"What is going on here?" Mother asked herself. "I know I've had arthritis and pains in the past, I never expected something like this. I am only thirty-six years old. I have children at home who need me. How is my husband faring without me? I want to go home. My hands and legs won't work. I can't go home. My family wouldn't know what to do with me." Then this poor mother cried.

As she lay there crying, she pleaded, "Dear God, please help me so I can go home and be with my children and husband. I know they need me so. I feel helpless. These seizures hurt something awful. God, please help me."

One day, the doctor came into her room and spoke quietly, "We have discovered your problem, Mrs. Deeker. You have a rare disease called Transverse Myelitus. I am sorry to tell you there is no known cure for this disease. It appears a virus attacked your spine which has debilitated you. We will do our best to give you good care. I am so sorry," the doctor continued as he patted her arm.

CHAPTER THREE

THEY CAN'T HELP ME?

"They can't help me?" Mother sobbed. "What do I do now?"

Mother lay suffering with seizures. Her fingernails would pierce into her hands and draw blood during a seizure. She was in agony each time her body cramped up. Her poor body was a victim to the virus that attacked her spine.

Week after week, month after month Mother lay there. She was not a complainer. In fact, she thanked the nurses for delivering her breakfast, lunch and dinner . She had to wait, sometimes a long time before a nurse had time to feed her the meal. Mother could not feed herself as her arms were totally paralyzed and lay limp.

Hour after hour this sweet Mother thought about her children at home. How was her baby boy? "He must be growing quickly," she said to herself. "I love those baby blue eyes and blond hair. His chubby cheeks are so kissable. I do miss them."

Tears rolled down her cheeks as she thought about her family back home. "God, please take care of my babies. They need their mother, but I can't take care of them. Thank you, God, for sending angels to look after my children."

"Hi mother," spoke Dorrie one day as she entered the hospital room. "What a beautiful bouquet of flowers," smiled Mother.

"They are from the garden. I am so happy to see you," smiled Dorrie as she kissed her mother's cheek. "We miss you so-o-o much at home."

"How are you doing, my dear girl?"

Dorrie spoke, "Oh Mother, I miss you so much. I can't keep the garden clean. I can't keep the house as clean as you kept it. We're eating the cookies so fast, I feel like I'm always baking."

"Do you get some help?" asked Mother. "Yes, Grandma comes over to help", said Dorrie, "but there is so much to do…..!"

"Yes my dear, it must be very hard for you. I wish I could help you," said Mother.

"Oh Mother," said Dorrie as she began to cry. "I was so-o-o hoping you would get better so you could come home. But look at your legs and arms. You can't even move them!" Dorrie buried her head in her mother's night gown and wept!

Papa soon appeared at the door and walked over to Dorrie. He stroked her hair and spoke. "It's alright Dorrie. We must go now so we don't tire your mother too much."

Dorrie wiped her tears and lingered at the bedside while holding her mother's hand.

Papa felt badly too that their fourteen year old daughter had so much work to cope with at home. He tried to help as much as he could by kneading the bread once a week. It was too big a job for the fourteen year old.

As Dorrie left her mom's hospital bed, she kissed her and then waved as she walked out the door. Papa gently kissed his wife and they chatted for a few minutes. Papa spoke, "Mother's Day is coming. I can bring the children to the hospital for Mother's Day. We will bring a picnic basket with a nice lunch."

Mother spoke, "I don't think I am well enough to sit in a wheelchair out on the grass." There was a lawn on the hospital grounds and Papa so wanted the family to be together. Mama said she would try to go outside that day.

On Mother's Day all the family were together on the lawn at the hospital. The children were delighted to see their mother. She tried to put on a brave front for the family as Dad wheeled her out of the hospital to the freshly cut green grass. The children were excited to see their mother, but they could also see that she was not doing well.

She smiled as each child gave her a hug. She said, "My, how you are all growing."

The family heartily ate their lunch, chatting away. An hour passed by and Father could see that his sweet wife was getting very tired. She was obviously slumping in her chair with her head down.

"I must take Mother back to her bed in the hospital," Dad spoke. "You girls clean up please and put everything back into the basket. I'll be back soon and we'll go home."

Each one kissed Mother goodbye. "Come home soon, Mommy. I love you, " they all whispered as Daddy slowly pushed the wheelchair toward the hospital. The six children watched their mother till Dad took her around the corner of the hospital. Could this be the last time the family was together? Would this be the last time the children would see their mother? Every day their mother got weaker and weaker!

"The most automated appliance in the household is the Mother."

CHAPTER FOUR

WHAT HAPPENED TO OUR ANGEL?

---Rrr i n gg Rrr i n gg Rrr r i n gg

"The telephone is ringing," called Beth, the second eldest daughter. The telephone had just been installed on the farm and the family was not used to this new gizmo.

"Hello," the children heard Dad speaking. It was 7.00 a.m. Who called that early in the morning, the girls questioned.

"Is this Jacob, Angela's husband? " the doctor asked.

"Yes it is," spoke Dad.

"I am sorry to tell you Mr. Deeker, that your wife died at 6:00 a.m. this morning," the doctor stated.

"What?" poor Daddy sobbed, "She's dead? It can't be – no-o-o it can't be!"

Life stood still for the family.

No one ate any breakfast that morning.

Grandma came over and helped the family where she could. She'd lost her eldest daughter. "What will this family do now?" she sobbed.

The cows needed to be milked and the chickens had to be fed. Several hours went by after that dreaded phone call. The farm animals called out. The cows mooed and the chickens clucked. The animals did not know that life as it had been for the Deeker family had come to a stand still. They had been hoping against hope that Mother would return home and things would be normal again. It was not to be.

Word soon got out, and neighbours came to help. Soon, there was a flurry of activity. The cows were milked and fed. The chickens settled down after they'd been fed and their eggs were gathered into the big yellow baskets.

Uncle John came over to help Dad plan the details for the memorial service and burial. What a painfully sad funeral service it was. To see this large family hovering around their mother's casket was extremely heartbreaking!

Poor Papa could hardly handle it! "What am I going to do"? he sobbed!

No doubt a piece of his heart died when his precious wife, lover, and friend died. Six children and no mother to share things with.

Friends, family and neighbors helped the family so much during the horrendous difficulties. This was greatly appreciated but who could replace this huge hole in the family???

"The help continued after Mother died. People were very good to the family but who could replace their kind gentle loving mother?" Heidi questioned . "Obviously, God needed another beautiful, caring and loving angel in Heaven so he took our mother.

"We know that each one of us will learn and become better as a result of this," said Heidi while a lonely tear ran down her cheek.

"I must tell you this one beautiful very special memory I will never forget! Mother and I were doing dishes. I was just four years old. Mother washed the dishes and I stood on a chair and dried them. We were chatting away and my mother made me feel totally cherished and very, very special as she hugged me.

"Her desire was to spend ten minutes each day per child and this was my ten minutes." She took that teaching moment to teach me how to dry the dishes well. She made me feel so loved and embraced in those tender moments!" spoke Heidi with a big smile on her face.

"I was only four years old when my mother died. Little did I know how these four short years could affect my young life! My wonderful mother left an indelible impression on me," spoke Heidi with excitement dancing in her eyes. "The four short years mother spent with me helped to give me the tenacity I needed in my challenging life."

Heidi spoke softly. "My doll was a very good friend to me. I remember the first Christmas after Mother died, my doll disappeared. I couldn't find her anywhere! I searched and searched and searched for her. I looked under my bed, searched through my messy closet and prayed to God to please help me find my doll."

This lovely little doll Rosey had the prettiest sparkling brown eyes that matched her cute curly brown hair. She wore a sweet lacy pink dress. Heidi cherished her so. She was truly her best friend! She talked to her and sang to her.

"I took her with me for a walk through the woods and together we'd admire the beautiful tall evergreen trees swaying in the wind. In Spring we'd admire the white and purple wild Easter lilies growing under the trees. There was a sea of colour – the plum coloured bleeding hearts, adorable little blue violets and purple trillium popped up here and there. I can't forget the bright yellow buttercups peeking their little heads amongst the foliage throughout the woods. This beautiful creation was so extravagant, my doll and I couldn't help but sing 'How Great Thou Art', a song I'd learned in Sunday School," revealed Heidi.

That was early December when Heidi had lost her best friend. Rosey. She continued to search all over, even in the hayloft where her two brothers and three sisters used to play a lot, but Rosey had disappeared.

The Christmas season was fast approaching. Heidi, together with her family, was busy baking and decorating cookies. Added to that, was rehearsing for Christmas concerts for school and church. For the time being, Heidi's mind was lost in the preparations for Christmas, though the thought of Rosey was always in the back of her mind.

Then came Christmas morning!

The children awoke early and bounded down the stairs. They ran into the living room and there stood the beautiful Christmas tree with all its decorations. Red and white bows were tied just below the white candles they'd lit the night before. Then there were gold and silver stars dotting the Christmas tree. The beautiful angel rested at the very top and she sang "Silent Night" while her head bobbed from side to side.

As Heidi glimpsed at the gifts so colourfully wrapped under the tree her eyes fell upon a pink doll cradle that rocked. She fixed her eyes on that cradle and WOW! - her name was on it! She fell to her knees in awe and was mesmerized for a moment!

"Oh! Oh! Oh!" Heidi cried. "Here is Rosey in her very own new bed, a pretty pink blanket and a new soft white night gown. She hugged Rosey so hard, She knew Rosey had missed Heidi as much as she'd missed her.

Papa had bought the cradle and Grandma had sewn the blanket and pretty white night gown for Rosey. Heidi knew Papa loved her dearly and so did her precious Grandma. Whenever Heidi could go and spend the night at her Grandma's house, she felt bathed in her love. What a treat! Her gentle Grandma was as loving and kind to her as her mother had been. The memories of these two dear people in her life helped her through a lot of challenges.

Speech-making is a bit like prospecting for Black Gold. If you don't strike oil In 10 minutes, stop boring.

CHAPTER FIVE

PAPA WAS VERY LONELY

Within a short time after Heidi's mother died, Dad felt ever so abandoned. Dad was lonely and had an urgent need to have a mother in the family. Heidi's Dad, being an extremely social individual, soon pursued some help for his need for a female companion.

Dad had a friend, Helen who was single. Two years after their mother's untimely death, Dad and Helen were married. Dad had been alone for ten lo-o-ong months while Heidi's mother was in the hospital. This poor man felt overwhelmed at this daunting task of raising six teenagers alone. One night Dad and Helen went out for a drive and Dad popped the question.

"Will you marry me, Helen?" Helen was shocked, because this question happened so quickly.

"I don't want to wait long," continued Dad. "The children need a mother, I need help. With teenage girls, I feel totally inept. Could you give me an answer in two weeks?"

Words could not describe how overwhelmed Helen felt. That evening, when Dad walked Helen to her door, she was quiet as Dad kissed her good night. Helen opened the door to her cozy apartment and stepped inside and shut the door.

Leaning against the closed door she sighed. "How can I ever step into Angela's shoes? She was such a good mom," Helen reflected. "I can't imagine, what it will be like to take over somebody else's teenagers. That man wants an answer in two weeks? That is madness," blurted Helen angrily as she mumbled to herself.

"I know I want to get married sometime, but to that man?" She thought to herself. "Yes, I am in my late thirties, so maybe if I want to have my own children, I'd better consider this offer seriously."

Helen threw herself on her bed and bellowed, "No, I won't."

Dad drove back to his house. "I'm not sure if this is the best decision but I'll make it work. The children like her. How bad could it be?" he asked himself.

Dad knew that, at times, he and Helen did not get along well, but he was desperate to have a companion.

Dad got home and thought, "Everyone is in bed and all is well. That's a good sign."

But it was not so.. Heidi's sisters had sneaked out and partied. Only Heidi and her two brothers were at home sleeping.

At 1:00 A.M. in the morning, Heidis sisters crawled through the basement window they'd left open. Then they quietly crawled up the creaky stairs.

Dad heard the noise, got up and snarled, "Who is that?"

The girls dared not breathe while they stood motionless. They held their breath till all was quiet again. They heard the snoring start. The girls, oh so stealthily, climbed another few stairs and then they stopped and listened.

Dorrie whispered to Beth, "I think we can continue now."

"That was close," whispered Beth as they slowly dragged their tired bodies up the stairs. They quietly tiptoed into the bedroom.

"Wasn't that fun tonight? I love to look into Harold's dreamy blue eyes," whispered fifteen year old Beth as she climbed into bed.

A few weeks later, Dad announced, "There is going to be a wedding, I am going to marry Helen."

"Oh my," wondered the children as they contemplated this announcement. Yes, they knew this pompous lady and wondered about the change this decision could bring about. They could only imagine!

The wedding and Christmas happened in the month of December. What a flurry of activity. It all happened so quickly!

Then came reality!

Everyone was greatly challenged to adapt to this totally new situation.

The children missed their mother very much! Their new mom had a completely different personality from their mother. Now this new wife of their dad lived in their home. She wasn't a special auntie dropping in from time to time. She used to love to say hi and bring treats..

Helen was a nurse by trade. She'd never had children and so the only way she knew to handle this challenge was to discipline the children with the paddle in anger and rage. Heidi was not impressed.

Heidi's father had been the disciplinarian before and now the children had two disciplinarians in the home. Gone were the familiar warm and tender hugs from their mother.

It wasn't long after the wedding, Heidi remembered waking up from a deep sleep, hearing her loving Dad embroiled in a loud argument with her step mom. The next thing she heard was the motor of a car driving away.

"Oh no," her little heart raced. "Is my Daddy leaving us now too?"

Her frightened, little six year old mind imagined the worst.

Heidi remembered how, due to the stress of the new situation, she started wetting her bed at night time.

This was a traumatic situation for everyone! Wetting the bed was just one symptom of the stress Heidi felt.

Going through the death of her mother, getting a new mom, and starting school were too many changes within a single year.. For Heidi, her body reacted.

Although Heidi was somewhat of a fragile child, there was much strength in her soul. She had the iron will and forthright manner from her father. She was also blessed with the warmth and gentle kindness of her mother.

Heidi was very chatty as a child. One of her teachers put tape across her mouth to keep her from talking with the student next to her. She was seven years old and loved her teacher. She had a hard time keeping quiet.

Through the years, friends of Heidi's folks loved to drive out to the farm from the big city of Vancouver. She remembers on one of these trips, the friends brought their 14 year old son, Franz with them.

He was a tall blond haired blue eyed young man. Franz sauntered around the yard and had been told that there was a cherry tree in the back forty. He could taste the sweet juicy cherries as he thought about the plump juicy cherries calling out to be devoured!

On the farm, the family had a beautiful large cherry tree with delicious cherries on it. The tree was shaped like a bride's dress, with a huge wide skirt! Heidi was swinging on the swing Papa made for their family when she noticed Franz.

"Hi," called Franz. "Do you have a cherry tree out here?" hurrying his step a little.

"We sure do!" spoke Heidi as she jumped off the swing, her blonde pigtails bouncing in the air.

"What's your name?" Franz questioned young Heidi.

"My name is Heidi," she responded. "Would you like to have some yummy juicy cherries?" asked eight year old Heidi.

"Would I ever," the young lad smiled. "Can you take me out there?"

"Sure can, come on," and the two started running through the pastureland where the cows grazed.

"I'll beat you," invited Heidi as she hurried along.

"You will not," called Franz as he picked up his pace.

Suddenly, there stood the cherry tree in all its beauty, beckoning them to come and taste of its bountiful harvest.

"Wow!" exclaimed Franz. "What a beauty."

"Try them," Heidi coaxed. "They truly are delicious."

It didn't take Franz long to pick cherry after cherry and pop them into his mouth!

Eventually, Franz put some cherries into a bucket and spoke. "Thank you very much for taking me out here, Heidi." He so enjoyed this excursion. It wasn't often he had a blissful opportunity like this!

After some time, they sauntered back to the big white farmhouse. "What a great day!" exclaimed Franz, "that was awesome."

I'm told that the best speech makers follow three simple rules. Stand up, speak up, then very quickly, shut up. I'll try to stick to that advice.

CHAPTER SIX

WHATAJOLT

Heidi was an average teenager who loved life.

Yes, life definitely had its challenges with a step mom on the scene.

Heidi felt close to her Dad. She knew he loved his family very much.

When she was sixteen years of age, her dad took her to get her driver's license.

Her mom was also in the car fussing and fuming about who knew? She was a very angry woman always upset about something. After listening to a constant battle between two adults on the way to Mom's work, Heidi stopped the car and let Mom get out of the car. This was her place of work. She was a very unhappy lady. Was her new role of being a step Mom too much for her?

Heidi continued driving down the road and Dad turned to her. "Be sure," he spoke, "that you marry the right person when you have to make that decision."

His message was loud and clear. He was very tired of listening to his wife's constant nagging. Heidi never forgot that advisement from her dad.

Within an hour, Heidi had her driver's license and she was whistling Dixie.

Heidi enjoyed playing sports at school.

On a lovely sunny afternoon, her gym class was out on the grassy field playing a game of softball. She was on third base and ran to home plate, trying to get there before the ball did. Running with all of her might, she slammed into the catcher who was a strong, sturdy girl. Thump! Her body groaned as she crashed to the ground.

She immediately picked herself up off the ground and dusted the dirt off of her white shorts and that was the end of the game.

She didn't remember feeling an injury after that ball game but she certainly felt some numbness on her right side before she'd walked a mile home to her house in the country. She had a limp and her right leg was dragging!

Within the following week, Heidi had term exams to write. By this time, her right hand was somewhat paralyzed. Her writing was difficult to decipher, but she handed the exam paper in. However, she knew she'd done poorly. Needless to say, Heidi failed her final exams that year. Something strange was happening to her body!

Her right leg limped when she walked, and at times fatigue took over her body to the point of complete exhaustion.

Her body acted strangely and the doctor had no answers.

The brain is a wonderful thing. It never stops functioning from the time you're born, until the moment you stand up to make a speech.

CHAPTER SEVEN

A TYPICAL TEENAGER

One evening Heidi and her friends attended a school party during her memorable last year of high school. Papa kindly let her borrow the car that evening to go to the party with her friends. She picked up her friends and drove a few miles out on the country roads. She found the big white house with blue shutters around the windows and knew that it was the place where the party was being held.

There were about twenty to thirty kids sitting in the barn when she and her friends got there. They were told that they were going on a hay ride. They soon climbed on the hay wagon. Some of the kids sat on hay bales. Heidi and her friends dangled their legs over the side of the wagon.

Soon they were served delicious hot chocolate which tasted warm and wonderful.

Suddenly, the horses jerked the hay wagon. The hot chocolate spilled down Heidi's white sweater!

"Oh, what a mess," she complained. Now she was embarrassed.

Soon they were on their way, the horses getting into a bit of a trot. What a jovial time they had on that hayride. They laughed hilariously as the trailer jostled through the pot holes in the road. They rode the hay wagon for about an hour.

They laughed so hard when the horses had to make a potty stop. Wow, did it stink!

"I'll tell you a joke," laughed Jerry, one of the guys at the party, and he began.

"Did you hear about the Texan? He had a huge ranch with thousands of horses on it. He also had a large swimming pool close to the house. Next to the swimming pool were tennis courts. About four times a year he'd invite all his friends to a party. Every year he invited his friends to go for a swim. In the pool," he said, "there was an alligator. Anyone who could swim the length of the pool without being bit by the alligator got one of three things. They would get half a million dollars, half of the estate, or the hand of the Texan's daughter.

No one ever took him up on his offer.

One evening, however, there was a lot of chatting and laughter going on. Suddenly, there was a splash! Everyone turned to look at the pool. There was a young man frantically swimming just as fast as he could.

Just as the alligator came dangerously close to him to rip off his leg, the swimmer quickly scrambled out of the pool. Panting breathlessly, he watched as the tall Texan strode through the crowd and stood next to the young swimmer.

'Very well done, young man,' drawled the Texan. 'Now what is your desire? Is it one million dollars?'

'No,' said the young man, 'It is not.'

'Then do you wish to have half of my estate?'

'No,' emphatically stated the handsome fellow, his piercing blue eyes fixed on the Texan.

'Ah, then it is my lovely daughter you are asking for? You desire her hand in marriage?'

'No, it is not,' stated the gentleman impatiently.

'Then what is it you want?'

'I want to know who pushed me in.'"

Everyone laughed heartily.

Soon after that, the horses pulled the hay wagon close to the barn.

"This was great fun," everyone exclaimed as they jumped off the wagon. "Thank you so much," they called to the farmer and waved goodbye and climbed into the vehicle.

On the way home from the party, Heidi was speeding on the quiet country road, showing off. A car with fellows from the party raced past her car. Being a wild sixteen year old, she increased her speed to follow the guys. The guys suddenly slammed on their brakes! With her inexperience in driving, even though she slammed on her brakes, it was too late. Suddenly there was a crash!

Her head bounced off the windshield! Heidi was stunned and saw blood dripping on her clothes.

"What should I do?" screamed Heidi, "I smashed my Papa's brand new red and white Impala!"

She was so mortified and wanted to hide in the ditch and not be found!

Heidi was filled with remorse.

Her Dad was so good to her and allowed her to have the car that evening. Because of her foolishness and stupidity, she wrecked his car. She felt wretched.

Heidi didn't know what happened after that.

The next thing she remembers is that she was at the hospital. It was there that the doctor sewed several stitches into her forehead to close the bloody, gaping gash.

Heidi knew she had no choice but to face the music from her Papa. It wasn't long before her father walked into the hospital to meet her. Heidi expected anger and rage as to what she'd done to her dad's brand new car! However, his compassion and kindness came through loud and clear. He looked at her with mercy and gentleness, not anger in his eyes.

"I am so very sorry, Dad", she blurted while bursting into tears. In his wisdom, he knew she'd had enough punishment!

He just looked at Heidi and spoke, "Let's go home".

Heidi has never forgotten her father's kindness.

She was expecting at least a tongue lashing which could have gone something like this: "I knew I shouldn't have allowed you to take the car tonight, especially because you were taking some friends with you. Why didn't you slam on the brakes when you saw the driver in front of you with his bright red brake lights on? What's the matter with you? Weren't you thinking?"

Obviously, Heidi had a very forgiving father.

Heidi had to go to Court. She felt terrified as she entered the court room. She felt like a criminal. The benches were cold and hard. The judge at the front of the room facing the court room sat very stoic and passionless. Heidi's hands shook and her voice faltered as she took the stand.

The judge asked her a few questions.

"Madame," the judge spoke. "Were you driving a 1964 Chevrolet Impala out on the country road that evening?

"Yes, I was." quietly answered Heidi.

"Were you speeding?" asked the judge.

"Yes, I was," answered Heidi as she hung her head.

"You are thereby charged with an offense of driving with undue care and attention causing an accident. You were also following a vehicle too closely! You must pay a fine of $75.00 to the courts."

"Ouch," thought Heidi. I only get $10.00 a month allowance, that'll take me some months to pay that fine!"

She was very fortunate in that her dad took care of the car insurance and never complained.

Why does a woman work for 10 years to change a man's habits, and then complain he's not the man she married?
– Barbara Streisand

CHAPTER EIGHT

LIKE JOSEPH? WORKING THROUGH PAIN AND HURT

Do you remember Joseph from the Bible? The chap whose dad favoured him and made him a coat of many colors? His many brothers taunted him more because of his new coat?

Why did his brothers' hate him? Did his father perhaps show more affection to this one child? Was there a special connection for this particular child?

Joseph and his younger brother Benjamin were, after all, the only offspring of beautiful Rachel. She was the gorgeous, dark haired, witty woman with stunning brown sparkling eyes. Was it because this lady was Jacob's first love – that their dad had a fondness for the two children from her, particularly Joseph, their firstborn?

Remember Joseph had a dream about his brothers who sincerely hated him. In this dream the brother's were all bowing down to him.

"How disgusting," the brothers mocked. "Who does he think he is? This stuff has really gone to his head! He's a lot worse since our father made him that crazy colorful coat. His d-r-r-e-a-m coat!" They scoffed! "How about that. What a nut! We'll show him!" they cajoled while they tended their father's sheep in the field.

It wasn't long before Joseph was sent out to the field to check on his brothers.

"Here comes the dreamer," they mocked as they saw him walking toward them from a distance.

"Let's kill him," one brother sarcastically shrieked! "Let's not do that,'" said another. "Let's sell him to the Egyptians in the chariot coming by."

Did Joseph often feel alone? He did have a younger brother named Benjamin. Joseph knew that he himself was not well loved by his older brothers. Especially after the dreams Joseph had and shared with his family, he, no doubt was much less respected by his older brothers.

Heidi felt lonely and afraid after she lost her mother. She cried and cried.

The new mom didn't realize the big shoes she had to fill and was in despair as time went on. Her life was constantly barraged with many interruptions throughout the day. Her need for companionship and time alone were not at all satisfied. Her personality did not delight in six individual temperaments who were constantly feeling their pain due to the loss of their mother.

Heidi's Dad and Helen were together because there was a huge hole in the family, not because they loved each other.

Consequently, Heidi felt very isolated as the hugs she'd always received from her mother were not there anymore. Heidi cringed as she thought of the trauma in the home. There were many insults, criticism and a lot of physical and emotional abuse.

Heidi felt like Joseph at times. She felt left out of the family many times, not feeling accepted as Heidi?

Maybe Heidi was different in that she cherished a special bond with her father?

Perhaps after losing her mother, there was much frustration and anger in the family.

"Was picking on one family member a coping mechanism?" Heidi questioned thinking to herself.

How do family members muddle through loss and loneliness? Is there perhaps a lot of tight fisted groveling going on due to fierce anger? Was the family left in a position where they did not know how to mourn their loss?

As a result, was there an inability to deal with the hurts of the past? The family struggled through life's horrendous challenges and had difficulty getting on with their lives in a healthy manner.

Sometimes, one can live in denial and have an unwillingness to think about one's pain. Is it possible to attend to the very feelings we so much try to escape?

Over time, Heidi worked through her pain. She loved to talk about her sweet mother! The tender memory of chatting and doing the dishes with this beloved, kind and gentle angel is forever etched in her mind.

"Mother made me feel very special," said Heidi softly.

Through mourning loves and losses are we able to deepen a personal relationship with ourselves and then connect better with other people?

Children are often very vulnerable, especially after they lose a parent.

Heidi felt a keen sense of rejection in her younger years. Due to the loss of the many affirming hugs and reassurances she had received from her mother, Heidi looked for love and acceptance from the older siblings. It was not forthcoming.

Consequently, there was a lot of fighting amongst the siblings. Slamming doors in anger, biting one another and slapping each other around. Was this a coping mechanism?

In time, Heidi learned that adversity happens in life, and life is a learning journey. Through journeying, she learns to share with others who are also looking for answers?

Now back to Joseph's story.

After the mean brothers sold Joseph to the Egyptians, Joseph spent time in prison, though he was innocent. He had not committed the crime for which he'd been wrongfully blamed. Potiphar's wife tried to force this seventeen year old to have sex with her. However, Joseph ran quickly from this evil lady. She then reported to her husband that young Joseph tried to force her to have sex with him.

Consequently, Joseph was sent to prison where he laboured for many years. He was a man of integrity. He was taught well by his father and endured suffering. He endured the test of time and humbly performed his duties.

In time, he became the ruler of Egypt! Then there was a famine in the far away land where his family lived and were starving. Who came to him for help in their time of need? Yes, the mean brothers. They begged Joseph on their knees for food. Little did they know who they were begging from. The dream Joseph had had as a boy was happening.

Little do we know how life will occur providentially. Here God sent Joseph on ahead. What the brothers meant for evil, God worked out for good. Those guys were so-o lucky!!

Heidi felt alone in her family as no doubt Joseph felt. Heidi however, had a real bond with her father. Was this a point of contention in the family? Joseph's brothers noticed a bond between Joseph and his father. Did this cause problems?

The trouble with being the best man at a wedding is that you never get to prove it.

CHAPTER NINE

GRADUATION AND THEN?

The year was 1969 and Heidi looked forward to her high school graduation! Heidi wondered who her escort would be at her graduation. She was looking around for someone who was not working or tied up that Friday evening.

One afternoon, in the month of May, friends of Heidi's parents happened by one day. These folk loved to drive out to the country from the city a few times a year. They loved to stop by and chat with Heidi's parents over a cup of tea.

Heidi rushed over to the settee where the adults were having tea, and chatted for a moment. "How is your son Franz? Where is he located at this point in time in his travels?"

"Oh," said the prestigious looking gentleman, "Franz has come home from the North and is now working in the big city."

As Heidi waved good day to the four adults and rushed out the door, she got to thinking, "This could be my answer. Here is an unattached young gentleman who has a job and a nice car. Maybe he could be my graduation date," Heidi thought to herself.

Heidi contacted Franz via a note with a school picture of herself tucked inside. When Franz received her letter, he was pleasantly surprised.

The reason was, Franz had recently backed out of an engagement to a girlfriend. Being newly single, he was pleased to "meet" someone new.

The night of the graduation he brought Heidi a lovely red rose corsage! Heidi was thrilled and giggled with delight.

The young man invited Heidi to spend the weekend in the big city and what a grand time they enjoyed. Franz planned with his friends to show Heidi a good time and show her the big city. Heidi grew up in the country so this was truly an adventure.

After the exciting graduation in the country Franz took Heidi home to her house to get a change of clothes before they were off to the big city.

Heidi wore a lovely white knee length taffeta gown with long lace sleeves to the graduation. She looked gorgeous. Her hair dresser made sure each hair was in place for this delightful occasion. Franz had his camera ready and took many pictures while Heidi smiled as she posed for him.

"I'll be right back," Heidi called over her shoulder as she ran off to change and pick up her overnight bag.

"What a great weekend this will be, he is such a sweetie!" Heidi thought to herself. It was an hour's drive into the big city but the time went so quickly as they chatted and laughed all the way.

"The lights are so beautiful!" Heidi was mesmerized as she watched in amazement! She was not at all used to a sight like this as they crested the hill over looking the city.

Franz soon found a little restaurant to have a bite to eat. It was now the wee hours of the morning, and Franz had a big day planned for Saturday. Together with some friends, Franz had a lovely picnic planned. He took Heidi to her friend, Amanda's house for the night. "See you tomorrow at 11:00 a.m." Franz called as he waved good-bye and drove off in his shiny new blue Convertible.

The next morning, after a good night's sleep at Amanda's house, Heidi was ready. Franz arrived on time. They smiled at one another with a good morning as Franz, the gentleman that he was, opened the door for Heidi who slid into the passenger seat. The next stop was to pick up Franz's friends, Jessica and Jerry. Within minutes, the party was complete with a lunch packed for the picnic and they were off.

Franz in the driver's seat, drove through the big city, over a long bridge and up and down many hills, snaking around many curves. After miles and miles of travelling through the mountains they came to a delightful picnic ground. The scenery was sublime!

There were orange and brown butterflies, and yellow and white butterflies, nesting on the flowers. All around them were majestic mountains dusted with a little snow. Nestled in the valley was a little Austrian like town. Talk about grandeur! Heidi was totally awed by the magnificence all around her! This day was so glorious that Heidi could hardly contain herself.

The two happy couples sat down at the table after Jessica and Jerry set the food onto the table. There was fried chicken, buttered rolls, potato salad, crunchy veggies and crispy apple squares for dessert. Everything was so delicious out in the fresh mountain air, thought Heidi. What a choice location they were enjoying with these very personable and kind friends of Franz .

Heidi was impressed and became more so as time went on. This Franz was truly amazing. First, the lovely corsage and perfume he'd presented for the graduation, and now the picnic in this enchanted setting.

As the afternoon wore on, they strolled up the mountain. Heidi so enjoyed the colourful foliage-purple, yellow, pink and lavender flowers waved in the gentle breeze.

Eventually it was time to head back to the city. Franz had a big evening planned and wanted Heidi to enjoy what was still to come. These two were beginning to really enjoy each other's company. Was this the beginning of a long journey ahead together?

That evening ,Franz entertained Heidi again to some fine dining and together they had a lovely romantic evening. The next day, Franz took Heidi home to the country with the promise that they'd see each other again soon.

The graduation was in the month of June. The following month July, Heidi moved to the big city to work. She settled in with a Jewish family as a nanny. Franz wanted her close by because he thought the drive into the country was too far every weekend.

Heidi was very happy to leave home as she'd reached the age of wanting her independence. Living closer to her special someone was truly a drawing card, and since Heidi was adventurous, she was delighted to make the move to the big city.

These two continued dating, and in six months there was a wedding!

Yes, this was the lad who, when he was fourteen, came out to the farm and eight year old Heidi led him to the cherry tree. Franz was a city boy, so the farm was a place he was not familiar with. The cows in the pasture frightened him, but eight- year- old Heidi knew her way around and she felt comfortable among the cows.

"Where there is a will, I want to be in it."

CHAPTER TEN

WEDDING BELLS

Heidi and Franz chose February 4th as their wedding day. It truly was a glorious day! Though it was raining, Heidi was deliriously happy. It was a February wedding, fittingly, their colors were red and white. The ceremony and reception happened at the little chapel in the wild wood. The countryside looked pristine.

The wedding party slowly drove through the valley honking their horns while everyone waved.

Family and friends wished them well.

After the reception Franz and Heidi rode off to pick up Franz' car which, Franz thought, he'd secretly hidden. Little did they know some 'one' thought they'd have some fun and discovered the 'secret' spot where the car was hidden.

Upon arrival, Franz immediately noticed the car was sitting very low. It didn't take long to discover all four tires had been flattened.

"Oh no," lamented Franz in disgust This is awful!! There are no service stations open at 11:30 at night, what are we going to do?"

After a minute or two Heidi spoke, "I have friends who own a service station, maybe they could help us."

Heidi and Franz had a friend Leslie, who had taken them to the 'hidden' car. Fortunately, he was still with the newlyweds when they discovered their dilemma. He was happy to help them, and kindly drove the newlyweds to Heidi's friend's house where the owner opened the door to their knock. The owner and his wife had been snuggled in their bed for the night, but after hearing the young couple's plight, were kind and helpful. After all four tires were pumped up, the car was ready to roll, and the newlyweds were on their way.

Their kind friend Jake, who helped them through this predicament, joked and laughed as he waved, "We mentioned you should come and see us, but we didn't expect you'd come so soon!" Franz and Heidi had a good laugh as they heartily thanked him for his generosity.

They thanked their driver Leslie, for taking the extra time to help them and then sped down the freeway to settle in to a comfortable hotel in Vancouver for the night.

The moon was low and the stars were out! They cruised on this journey with a very loud shout! What a blissful ride they enjoyed that night as they snuggled and cuddled together so tight!

The following day, Franz and Heidi sailed off to Victoria for an extravagant honeymoon weekend. As they sailed to Vancouver Island, Heidi and Franz so enjoyed the waves while viewing the picturesque mountains. The white snow glistened and sparkled under the warm sun that day. Hand in hand, and arms around each other, they bathed in their wild fabulous love. The kisses and hugs continued, as the two love birds sauntered around on the deck of the ship. This was heaven!

The ship soon docked in Victoria where the young couple slipped into their vehicle and drove off to find their honeymoon hotel.

The following day they dined extravagantly in a lavish but cozy Victorian like-old English teahouse! It was marvelous and wonderful. The teahouse was built on the waters' edge. Franz and Heidi enjoyed the splendour of the sparkling ocean with the majestic mountains in the distance!

It was a marvelous honeymoon weekend! They walked along the water's edge hand in hand. Heidi had never experienced life like this. They laughed and chatted as they strolled.

"This is my best friend," Heidi thought to herself. "This is the beginning of our new life together."

After four romantic days, it was time to set up their suite. They sailed to the mainland continuing their frolicking. They roamed around the ship again, singing this song:

You are my Sunshine, my only Sunshine,

You make me happy, when skies are grey

You never know dear, how much I love you

Please don't take my sunshine away.

The ship soon docked and the happy couple drove off to their new home. It was a cozy basement suite. It had a warm fireplace in the living room.

The first evening they were home Franz had to go to work. He kissed Heidi goodbye, "see you later," he sweetly whispered.

Heidi turned into her kitchen after she'd shut the door. "What will I do first?" she asked herself.

Heidi started with the pretty new yellow bath mat set for the tiny bathroom. They'd also got a blue set for a wedding gift. There were white bath towels with blue flowers. Another matching towel with pink flowers.

"This is like playing house with my best friend," Heidi thought to herself. She had so much fun setting the new linens in the cupboards. Then there were the pretty white and gold dishes to set on the table with cutlery. Heidi set the table for breakfast as she wanted to impress her love.

"In the morning, I'll make him a lovely tasty breakfast with eggs and pancakes," Heidi thought to herself.

After some time, Heidi was getting weary and wanted to climb into bed.

She turned toward the bedroom and realized the bed needed sheets and pillows. She soon found the pink Queen sized sheets, took them out of the package together with the pillowcases and made the bed. The western style romantic music played in the background while Heidi crawled into bed.

"Ah," she sighed, "I will awake to my lover at my side." Franz was due to come home from work at 2:00 a.m. after he'd completed his shift. Heidi soon fell asleep.

Light travels faster than sound. That is why some people appear bright until you hear them speak.

CHAPTER ELEVEN

THEIR TROUBLES BEGAN?

Three months after their wedding, Heidi came down with a painful bladder infection. Antibiotics were prescribed and the infection disappeared, or so they thought. Two months later, Franz and Heidi took a two-week honeymoon vacation to California. Two days after they left home, Heidi came down with a serious kidney infection. Franz's good friends in Portland, Oregon, where they stayed the night, suggested Heidi visit their excellent doctor.

The doctor was very kind and prescribed another strong dose of antibiotics medication. He also recommended that Heidi drink lots of cranberry juice. She followed the doctor's orders and the newlyweds were on their way again. Little did Heidi or Franz know that this was the beginning of an arduous, puzzling journey.

Their vacation to California was delightful. When they approached the desert of Palm Springs, the heat was unbearable! They dashed from their air conditioned vehicle into the cool ice-cream parlor where they cooled their tongues with a strawberry ice-cream cone.

Franz and Heidi started a tour up the mountain when their car decided it couldn't handle the heat. The radiator began angrily steaming, spewing out ominous sounds? Franz knew he'd better turn the car around and head back down the steep mountain. Their little car thanked them for that!

The couple soon knew they'd be more comfortable back in the Los Angeles area where it was cooler. Comfortably cooler.

They visited the San Diego Zoo, then on to Disneyland. What a delightful time they had!

War does not determine who is right – only who is left.

CHAPTER TWELVE

THE JOY OF CHILDREN

Within a year and a half of married life, Franz and Heidi were blessed with a darling baby daughter. She was gorgeous; she had curly blond hair and the most beautiful blue eyes. They had so much fun with this sweet little girl.

When Denise was nine months old, Heidi went through a six week period of blurry vision every evening. Perhaps it was due to fatigue she thought. After a good nights' sleep, the blurry vision disappeared.

"What was this all about?" Heidi questioned. Life continued on. They had a lot of living to do!

Two years later, they were blessed with an active little boy. He also had the blondest hair and baby blue eyes. He was only seven months old – Heidi was so-o-o-o tired, but what could she expect?

"No doubt it was due to having two little ones," Heidi reasoned.

Heidi went to see the doctor again. This seemed to be an event which was occurring too often. "Yes, you are going to have another baby!" the doctor announced. Within seven months Heidi and Franz had another blondie with the brightest blue eyes. She was also a gorgeous child.

With the third pregnancy, Heidi was so fatigued she could hardly do anything. She didn't know what her problem was. Two friends came over during that time and kindly cleaned her house for her. How blessed she was! God truly sent angels into her life to help her. That bout of total debilitating fatigue lasted two months It was an extremely difficult time for Heidi.

Heidi continued to suffer with severe fatigue. "No doubt," she convinced herself, "It's because I have three little children. They are a lot of work and were born so close together. "

Heidi also suffered with bladder infections off and on as well as a kidney infection which was very painful. The kidney infection lasted a year, during which time the doctors found the problem and she had major surgery. The urologist discovered after many tests, that she had no one way valves at the bottom of her ureters(a duct that carries urine from the kidneys to the bladder).

These valves allow the urine to pass from the kidney to the bladder and then they close so the urine can not go back up into the kidney. It was discovered that Heidi was born without these valves and it was not until after she was married did this problem manifest itself. With modern science, the specialist was able to make these valves using Heidi's own tissue, and to this day the new valves are still working.

"Yes, Heidi explains," I have to keep warm and be sensitive to bladder infections, but that is part of the arduous journey of my life."

Overcoming major surgery like that took a long time. Again a dear friend, Sylvia, came to spend a week with her to help look after the children. Another angel for which she was extremely grateful.

Franz was loving, and tried to be understanding. Heidi was totally stressed.

She could not understand why she was constantly suffering with severe fatigue. As a result, her specialist who'd performed the surgery, suggested that Franz take Heidi away on a week's vacation.

Franz's family were extremely compassionate, and took the children for that week. While they were away from home, Franz made sure Heidi ate healthy food and demanded she rest a lot.

That week was truly a week of respite. She had time to rebuild her body with good nourishing food and relaxation.

Franz was wonderful, and made sure she ate the best nourishing food which he cooked, and she enjoyed.

Little did Heidi know what a challenge she was struggling with. Little did she know what lay ahead! Was there a beast attacking her body?

There were good days! But there were bad days.

It was a difficult time for the children. They could not understand why they had to be without Mommy and Daddy for a week. They were very little. Their ages were one, two and four. Why were they in strange beds at night? They were terrified. They were in a caring, loving home but there were four big brothers. The brothers teased them mercilessly. They cried and cried, waiting for Mom and Dad to come get them.

Poor kids. It was an emotionally difficult time for everyone.

Their parents returned, and what a delight! Now they were together again.

One Sunday afternoon, Franz and Heidi took the family on a picnic. What a gorgeous view they enjoyed. They sat at the picnic table overlooking a gorgeous placid lake. In the distance were snow covered mountains. This was God's beautiful creation.

"This has to be the most beautiful place on this earth," they chatted as they feasted on their lunch.

They had tasty chicken with freshly buttered rolls. There were carrots and celery sticks to munch on. For dessert, there was an apple crumble.

"Yumm", the children smacked their lips as they lifted the spoons to their mouths. "Mummy, this is so-o good."

As they enjoyed their lunch, they listened to the birds singing in the trees. The squirrels scurried around the table at their feet to pick up crumbs from the ground.

After they'd licked their lips, they packed the picnic basket with the dirty dishes. Franz set the basket into the trunk of the car and the family were off for a hike.

They hiked down the hill toward the lake and over a short bridge. They watched the water cascade over the rocks in the creek as they crossed the bridge.

Suddenly, Heidi fell! For whatever reason, she had tripped. Her leg wasn't listening to her brain signals and she went sprawling. She quickly picked herself up off the ground and the family continued their walk.

"Ouch," complained Heidi. She held her second smallest finger on her left hand carefully. Franz looked at her finger compassionately for a few minutes, saw no blood and they continued hiking. Heidi's finger was sore for a year after that-perhaps a sprain happened as she fell.

Evening News is where they begin with 'Good Evening,'
and then proceed to tell you why it isn't

CHAPTER 13

HEIDI HAD FUN

Though she'd blamed her walking and falling problems on her sports injury for many years, a chiropractor was able to straighten out her spine. This treatment helped to bring healing to the body so the oxygen could flow more freely. Heidi walked a little better from the treatment.

Heidi had learned in her early thirties that staying off dairy products and watching her sugar intake was extremely helpful.

"Staying off sugar and dairy helped me beyond a doubt," spoke Heidi.

Her walking improved a great deal. Eating more vegetables than fruit helped her body, given there was too much sugar in fruit for her body to cope with. One to two fruits a day sufficed for Heidi.

Heidi loved her kids dearly and, recalled many of their childhood antics. Denise and Donny are the two eldest. With the blondest hair and the sparkling blue eyes they charmed their way to your heart. On one particular occasion they were walking home from school, and got into a scrap.

M. Joy (Willms) Neufeld

The rule in Heidi's house was to eat all your lunch. The kids had cheese whiz or tuna fish sandwiches every day. The kids got very tired and bored of this fare. On their way home from school one day, Donny decided to throw his yucky sandwiches into the forest.

There were many bushes at the side of the road the kids passed on their way home from school.

Denise said to Donny when she saw him throw his sandwiches away, "I'm going to tell on you and you'll get into serious trouble!"

Just about that time, Donny saw a snake slithering oh so quickly through the grass and under the bushes. With his agile feet, he quickly stepped on it. Then he grabbed its tail and picked it up. The snake writhed angrily in desperation while sliding his tongue in and out of its' mouth. He craved to get away from Donny's clutch. Donny held on and started chasing Denise with the snake. Denise screamed and ran as fast as her legs could carry her!

"I'll get you if you tell on me," called Donny as he chased Denise. They ran down the road after each other with Donny holding the writhing snake.

"Drop that stupid snake," screamed Denise as Donny got closer to her.

"Only if you promise not to tell on me," blurted Donny as he got closer to Denise.

"Drop it or I'll throw a rock at you and hurt you!" angrily shouted Denise as she picked a sharp rock up off the road.

They were both panting as they spoke and Donny blurted, "Okay, okay, I won't throw this snake if you don't tell!"

Denise backed away as she threw the rock on the ground. "Promise? Throw the snake away now," begged Denise as Donny reluctantly threw the snake into the bushes.

"Whew, I'm glad that's gone," spoke Denise as she breathed a sigh of relief.

They continued their walk home from school and in time, I heard the story. Kids will be kids..

Heidi's family went on a camping trip with their fun loving beautiful kids. Before they left home, a friend gave them a big box of fruit.

"Won't this be a delicious feast! We all really enjoy fruit," spoke Heidi to herself. There were luscious green and purple grapes. There was a honeydew melon and a cantaloupe. Added to that were apples and juicy oranges. The family were driving through the mountains with their trailer in tow while enjoying the horn of plenty with all its fruit.

As the family continued on their trip, the anxiety Heidi experienced was horrendous! Little did Heidi know how too much sugar could affect her mind!

She didn't know what to do.

She wanted to scream or spit or do something crazy! WHY? WHY? WHY?

She managed to control herself but what was going on? Heidi wanted to run away!

The family reached their destination. They found a beautiful campsite on the lake in the Okanagan! A desert-like area beside a gorgeous placid lake. People were swimming and boating, laughing and splashing each other.

Franz carefully backed the trailer onto the specified campsite.

"Stop," Heidi yelled.

"Now go forward three feet," continued Heidi.

"Get out of the way, kids," hollered Franz in his frustration. Phew, once again it was parked for a week.

They set up camp. The kids loved camping. Franz pulled their bikes off the trailer and off they rode. The kids really enjoyed swimming in the lake. They'd sit around the campfire at night and roast marshmallows. A great time was had by all.

They met wonderful neighbours that particular camping trip and these folks introduced them to a product known as Aloe Vera juice. This healthy juice has healing properties for the body. Due to the unhealthy acidic content of many bodies, including Heidi's, the Aloe Vera juice brought her body to a more healthy alkaline level. For ten years Heidi drank that juice. She also stayed off sugar and dairy products and her health improved beyond a doubt.

One day Franz did some research in The Columbia University College of Physicians and Surgeons Complete Home Medical Guide. Here he found pertinent information. He discovered that the prolonged medication Heidi had been on for infections could damage the immune system.

Heidi continued to read and apply remedies to her situation of severe fatigue.

Heidi learned about giving herself an enema to clean toxins out of her body. She thought, "I'll try it to help my body get some relief."

One day she locked herself in the bathroom. "This is the day," she said to herself.

"My own privacy, this is bliss." She felt she had very little time to herself. With three little ones, her own time was difficult to find.

Suddenly, there was a soft knock on the door. "Mommy, where are you?"

Heidi thought, "Oh no, no privacy."

"Go see your dad," she spoke to her daughter. Off Charlene went to play with her toys. She just wanted to know where her mommy was. Bless her little heart.

Heidi continued her procedure and discovered she truly did have more energy after her enema. The toxins in her body had been dragging her down. Removing toxins was s-o-o-o important to help her feel a little better-a little stronger.

"Now I have enough energy to keep up with our toddlers for a short while," said Heidi.

A bus station is where a bus stops. A train station is where a train stops. On my desk, I have a work station.

CHAPTER 14

KIDS DO GROW UP !

It seemed that the children raced through their formative years. They all graduated from high school and then went off to college.

In time the three found marriage partners.

"As the saying goes," says Heidi, "first comes love, then comes marriage, then comes along a baby carriage. Yes, there are eight wonderful grandchildren. What a delight! Family is so important and Heidi feels greatly blessed!"

"When the new babies, our grandchildren were born, I was hesitant to pick up these precious jewels as encouraged to by the babies' mother. My legs felt very weak and I didn't trust my legs to have the strength to stand while I held or carried these precious little ones. Thank God I never dropped a baby or fell when I was carrying one of these jewels, but I felt anxious about it.

I didn't want to disappoint my children and am so grateful the little ones were okay. I did not wish to express my uneasiness to my children but perhaps I should have. I know they would have understood. I wanted to be strong!"

One morning, Heidi was having a very good day. As she got on with her day, she said to herself, "I am going for a long walk today. I am sure I can handle it." The day was beautiful and sunny!

Heidi walked along the sidewalk singing away.

She had walked about a mile when her legs said, "We can go no further."

Heidi knew she could not go any further and sat down on the curb for a half hour. She didn't know how long she'd sit there. It could be a while before her legs would be strong enough to walk back home.

Cars kept driving by. Heidi thought to herself, "This must look hilarious to those folk driving by. Here I am, a middle aged woman sitting on the curb."

Suddenly, Heidi noticed a car driving by, it soon turned around and drove by very slowly. The driver stopped and kindly asked, "Do you need help?"

Heidi explained that she had to rest till her legs were ready to walk again.

The dear lady asked, "Would you like a ride?" Heidi responded, "I would so appreciate that."

She got into the car and the lady took her home. Another kind angel God brought Heidi that day. The lady was a nurse and asked Heidi questions about how long she'd had this problem? Heidi responded with, "I've had this problem for some time but the doctors have no answers."

No doubt she went home with questions in her mind after she dropped Heidi off.

I thought I wanted a career. Turns out I just wanted pay checks.

CHAPTER 15

AM I GOING BLIND?

It was October of 1996. Heidi awoke that morning to what she thought was a normal beautiful sunny day. Franz went off to work and Heidi began her routine. It wasn't long and she was fatigued and sat down on the couch to watch television.

She soon noticed black spots in front of her eyes. Before long she was seeing double as she watched the television.

"This is strange," spoke Heidi to herself. "I'm sure I'll be fine after a good nights' sleep."

The next morning, nothing had changed, so she went off to see the optometrist.

"Is there something I can help you with?" inquired the optometrist as he tested Heidi's eyes.

"Yesterday morning I awoke feeling alright. By the middle of the morning, while I was watching T.V., I saw black spots on the screen. Shortly after that I was seeing double."

"You must go to the hospital!" the doctor insisted. "This is something I cannot help you with!" he emphatically declared.

Heidi left the office and pondered, "I have no pain or blood, etc. Oh well, I guess this is another strange action in this weird body of mine. When Franz gets home we'll go to the hospital!"

At the hospital, Heidi was told to go see an ophthalmologist-this eye specialist soon identified the problem as a virus.

While testing her eyes, the kind doctor questioned, "Have you lost the taste in your tongue or do you have numbness in the face?"

"I have no problems there," replied Heidi.

"Then it's a virus and it will disappear in approximately six weeks."

"Six weeks?" thought Heidi to herself. It will not take six weeks! Heidi was determined her eyes would not take that long to revert back to normal.

She did not drive her car for a week as she felt it was safer not to. Heidi tried to busy herself while pondering what was happening to her.

In time, Heidi learned she could drive the car with double vision by placing a patch over one eye. She found parking the car was the most difficult for her as depth perception and distance was a challenge with only the sight of one eye.

Two months after the double vision began, the vision corrected itself.

Heidi had a question and proceeded to see her doctor once again. While sitting in the waiting room waiting for her name to be called, the pretty tiny dark haired receptionist called her name.

"Heidi."

She put her magazine down and followed the receptionist into the little stark office. She had gorgeous brown eyes. Heidi sat down on a comfortable chair and waited for the doctor.

The doctor entered the room and asked, "Any problems today?"

"I have weird tinglings jumping all over my body sporadically. I'm sure it's nothing."

The doctor looked at Heidi rather startled and began. "You are going to see a neurologist! First you had the double vision and now the tingling."

He immediately alerted his nurse to make an appointment with the neurologist just as quickly as possible. This was an emergency!

Heidi had the tingling for some time but felt it was just another of those mysterious sensations for this strange body of hers. She hadn't been alarmed about the tingling but decided to question the doctor, thinking he may have a quick simple explanation for her. This was not the case.

Within a few weeks, Heidi went to see the neurologist and his kind gentle manner put her at ease immediately. Through the years, Heidi had been to many doctors with extreme fatigue, stiffness in the legs and much trouble walking. Heidi so appreciated this doctors' compassion.

Heidi had been through some rather rude experiences with doctors and was not particularly fond of another doctor's questions and probes. By this time, she sensed that perhaps she'd get some answers and it could be worthwhile to go for more tests.

Within a short time, Heidi visited a neurologist. This doctor was so congenial and understanding. He was shocked that this was the first time she'd been to visit a neurologist.

The neurologist expressed, "I will be testing for Multiple Sclerosis as well as other problems. Among other tests you will be going to the Royal Columbian Hospital for an MRI – Magnetic Resonance Imaging – scan."

Heidi was not surprised to hear his comments as almost twenty years before this, she personally wondered if this was her problem. She questioned her doctor at that time, as she was suspicious that she may have MS.

After making this suggestion to her doctor, he rudely replied, "You do NOT have MS".

Heidi was in tears at this point and he continued harshly, "What's the matter with you? Do you have stress in your marriage?"

No doubt he thought this was a ridiculous idea! Consequently, Heidi ran from his office crying, feeling still more stressed. She never visited that doctor again.

Needless to say, she sought alternative therapy. Heidi constantly sought the best supplements she knew of to give her body more energy. The extreme fatigue was so debilitating!

Why was there constant stiffness in her legs? Why did she have balance problems and falling at times? Why could she not walk very far-she always got so tired. Her legs did not behave as she would have liked them to. Why, why, why?

After the tests were completed, the doctor called Heidi into his office. "The tests have proven that you have Multiple Sclerosis," stated the neurologist.

"You could continue to have attacks off and on or you may stabilize. We'll find you a neurologist at the UBC Hospital in Vancouver."

Heidi was forty-nine years of age when she was diagnosed with MS.

The doctors did not have a whole lot of answers to help MS so Heidi continued with her holistic, natural way of helping her body cope. She was very proactive.

Heidi thanked the doctor and left his office. She called Franz immediately to tell him the news. Now there was a diagnosis and they had something to work with.

In time, Heidi went to see another naturopath because her legs were so bad. She continued to have difficulty walking.

She spoke to herself, "Unless my legs improve, I'm going to be in a wheelchair."

Heidi had learned, diet made a huge difference and she continued with her program. She was in her early thirties when she learned about diet changes.. Although she had days of severe fatigue, she could keep going and live more of a "normal life".

Heidi's walking greatly improved when she went off dairy products as well as sugar.

She pursued living that way for ten years. It's not that Heidi never cheated, but worked very hard at eating what was best for her.

Heidi told me that, because she felt so much better, giving those things up was not a sacrifice.

After ten years of watching her eating habits, Heidi decided to eat like normal people and enjoy sugar and dairy. Within a very short time, she knew her health was deteriorating. She told herself, "I'm enjoying my food and I'll be okay. I'll live with whatever I have to."

Every so often, Heidi had a fall. Only once did she have to go to the hospital and have a few stitches put into her forehead. She got out of bed one afternoon, after having a nap, and Heidi fell. As she was walking out of her bedroom toward the hallway, Heidi lost her balance and her head hit the corner bead of the wall. Down she went!

Soon she saw bright red blood dripping on the blue grey carpet. Heidi refused to turn her head up because she didn't want the blood to drip into her eye.

Heidi called Franz who hurried upstairs from the basement. He looked at Heidi and was startled when he saw the bright red blood dripping on the floor. Franz hurriedly drove Heidi to the hospital where she was soon taken care of.

The doctor looked at the half inch cut and called the nurse to bandage it. Now Heidi felt much better. No scar was left. The bandage held the skin tautly together. WOW!

Over time, Heidi started using a cane for walking to stabilize herself. No doubt Heidi felt self conscious about the cane in the beginning. Over time however, she became aware of the necessity of the cane for safety reasons.

At times Heidi also used the wheel chair. Sometimes the fatigue was overwhelming. In order to go out Heidi needed the wheel chair and her husband pushed her around. Particularly in airports Heidi couldn't handle the walking and was so grateful for a wheelchair.

I didn't say it was all your fault, I said I was blaming you.

CHAPTER 16

NEVER TRUST A SLEEPING DOG

It was a glorious Tuesday morning in May of 1995. Heidi's friend Pat was joining her for lunch that day. Heidi stepped into her red convertible and drove to her friend's house to pick her up. Heidi knew her friend Pat had a dog, Dexter, but Heidi had no reason to fear this animal, she thought to herself.

As Heidi pulled her convertible onto the driveway, Heidi noticed the dog lying placidly on the concrete, his head resting on his paws as if asleep.

After parking her car on Patty's driveway, Heidi stepped out of the car and walked confidently toward the dog who was chained to the door knob. As Heidi lifted her foot toward the first stair, the dog barked ferociously and lunged at Heidi, sinking his sharp teeth into the calf of her left leg. Heidi turned to run. Due to the stiffness in her legs she promptly fell and her body smashed onto the concrete.

Heidi lay there limp and immobile!

Dexter continued to bite at her ankles as he barked. The dog could stretch his chain far enough to gnaw at her ankle as Heidi lay there moaning.

Suddenly, Patty was at the door! She quickly grabbed Dexter and locked him in the basement!

"Oh Heidi, I am so sorry!" Patty cried as she tried to help Heidi onto her feet.

"Leave me alone," moaned Heidi. She lay there in agony while her body tried to relax. It took some time before Heidi got the inner strength to lift her body off the concrete. With Patty's help, she slowly limped into the living room where Heidi lay down on the soft green couch.

"Please call Franz," requested Heidi. "He will take me to the hospital."

Slowly Heidi lifted her pant leg to survey the damage.

It wasn't long and Franz arrived. He heard the story and then helped Heidi to her feet. Hanging onto Franz, she hobbled to the car. Together, they drove to the hospital.

By this time, Heidi relaxed somewhat. Franz parked the car and helped Heidi as she limped into the hospital. The doctor was summoned. The doctor spoke and had some questions. Heidi needed a tetanus shot and the nurse promptly walked into the next room to get the needle. Swiftly, the nurse gave Heidi a tetanus shot.

The doctor examined the wounds. Yes, there was blood but they were only flesh wounds. She didn't need stitches. The kind nurse cleaned the wounds and after some time, Franz and Heidi returned home.

"Never trust a sleeping dog," exclaimed Heidi!

A clear conscience is the sign of a fuzzy memory.

CHAPTER 17

MENTAL AND EMOTIONAL FATIGUE

Having an illness has a profound effect on one's identity as a person. Not only does the individual have to deal with constant fatigue and limitations, but also the neurological effects. One's whole identity as an individual is tightly connected with how they feel about themselves.

Because Heidi has been extremely active in searching for answers to best help herself, she is still mobile.

It has been a very challenging journey for Heidi. She ravenously sought after support! Her wonderful husband has been there for her every step of the way. Their children often cannot understand what is going on, but love her through it all. She has good friends too, who have been there for her.

Heidi sought out counsellors, mentors, etc. to assist in her challenging journey of life.

Because Heidi has a very positive attitude and keeps searching for answers, she is a winner. For Heidi, denial is not part of her vocabulary. Because she suffered with a sports injury in high school, she always blamed her limp on the injury. That was when her right leg started dragging and she had partial paralysis on the right side of her body.

Heidi lets people know she has Multiple Sclerosis. She feels that takes the mystery out of her disabilities. She tries very hard not to burden people with her disabilities.

"Sometimes perhaps, folks tire of me when I sound like a complainer. One of my biggest challenges has been to stay with my healthy way of eating. We as a couple are very social and yes, I yield to temptations. Food is so-o tasty," laments Heidi.

Heidi keeps active. She is constantly aware of overdoing life and getting so fatigued that her zest for life is gone.

"I choose to be overly cautious. That way I can enjoy the next day if I get a good night's sleep."

For some people, the MS puts them into a wheelchair. Heidi finds that if she eats the right food, lots of raw vegetables with a balance of carbohydrates and fats, she can walk better. Exercise is extremely important as Heidi continues to learn. Part of the learning curve is not to stretch the body beyond its limits.

Attitude is huge! Don't worry-be happy!

To fight depression, here is a list of helpful remedies Heidi is learning to live by:
For anyone with depression, she suggested they try these remedies.

1. needs to be with people that appreciate you

2. be interested in feelings as well as logic

3. Take time for complex decisions

4. Needs time alone or with one or two others

5. Cannot be over scheduled

If there is too much stress, Heidi tends to withdraw, feel fatigued, indecisive, be pessimistic or overly sensitive to criticism.

A great thing to do in group situations Heidi is learning, when she feels stressed, she needs to practice talking casually with others and stay near the centre of the action. As stress can bring on fatigue,

Heidi is learning to relax while being more outgoing and involved in group situations.

Here is a list of suggested stress releases that Heidi recommends;

a. prepare yourself for big holidays or hectic social periods by spending more time being quiet and alone

b. set aside one weekend a month to be alone with that special person in your life. The more difficult that is to do, the more important it is to do.

c. You need solitude to recharge, so set a quiet time aside each day.

d. be proactive to avoid interruptions when you are working on a stressful task.

e. Keep a list of your recent successes and re-read it when you feel discouraged

f. Be sure you take time to have casual exchanges with your superiors

g. Reward yourself by doing things you always feel good about afterwards

You do not need a parachute to skydive. You only need a parachute to skydive twice.

CHAPTER EIGHTEEN

THANK YOU FRANZ!!!!

Over the years, Franz has been there for Heidi. She is so grateful to Franz for the kindness he has shown. Heidi thanks Franz for all of these things:

"Though life-marriage has been very difficult, it is the best and hardest decision I've made," speaks Heidi.

THANK YOU FRANZ- WHERE DO I START?

Thank you for loving your family so much!

Thank you for taking the family camping many times, we all had so much fun.

Thank you for taking the family to Disneyland two times.

Thank you for being there through the years, for holding my hand when we walked together. Then for going to get the car when I could not walk anymore and coming to pick me up as my legs gave up.

Thank you for filling my gas tank again and again.

Thank you for understanding when I was too tired to go out even when we'd just planned an outing and had to stay home.

Thank you for being romantic-for bringing me flowers on Mother's Day, Valentine's Day, Easter, etc.

Thank you for wanting to work at improving our relationship. I am so blessed that you want to put effort into building our marriage.

Thank you for genuinely caring.

Thank you for your commitment to marriage.

Thank you for finding dating an important part of the marriage.

There have been many difficult times for Heidi.

With illness, life can be extremely challenging in a marriage. Problems are compounded, misunderstandings happen quickly when assumptions are made.

THIS IS TRUE LOVE!!

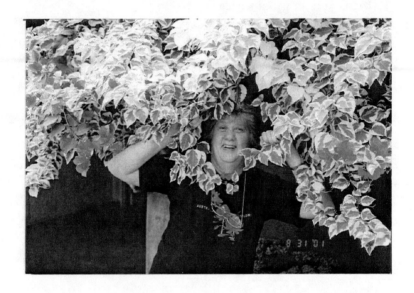

Heidi peeking through the tree in Hawaii

TO THE WOMAN I'M SO GLAD I MARRIED

I'm a better man
Because of you__
Lifted by your enthusiasm
Strengthened by your support,
And constantly renewed
By your love--------
You make all the difference
In my life,
And I couldn't have married
A more wonderful woman
Than you
HAPPY BIRTHDAY I LOVE YOU
F R A N Z

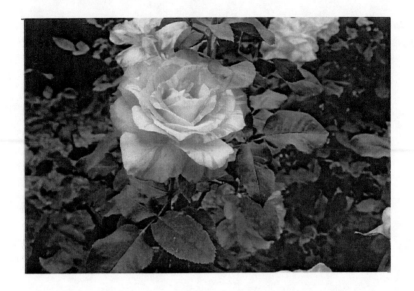

FOR MY BEAUTIFUL WIFE, YOU MAKE ME SO HAPPY!!

If I counted all the ways I've fallen in love with you through the years,
If I gathered each smile, each moment and memory that has brought
me true happiness,
And then somehow found the words that matched my feelings------------
Then you would always know that the only thing more wonderful than
Falling in love with you is, without a doubt,
    Living in love with you!

    With all my heart   HAPPY ANNIVERSARY!

            FRANZ

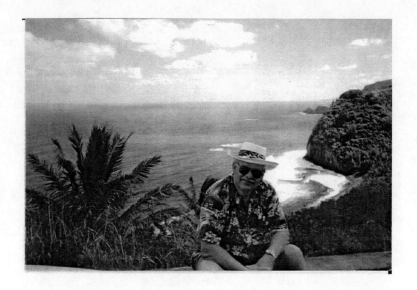

Franz sitting at the beach in Hawaii

Money can't buy happiness, but it sure makes misery easier to live with.

CHAPTER TWENTY

"HOW DID YOUR ILLNESS AFFECT THE CHILDREN?"

"I'm so glad you asked. Here is a heartfelt description of how our eldest daughter felt about the Multiple Sclerosis. It truly was hard on her. Denise wrote this, bless her heart.

"Growing up with a family member who has MS is a huge struggle for everyone involved. When it's a mom, it seems to have a larger impact, at least that has been my experience. Mom's are nurturing beings, and when they cannot operate in that capacity, it has an affect on everyone. First off, growing up, we had no idea what was wrong with our Mother. We just knew she slept a lot. The second thing is, as I was the oldest child, it felt like a lot of things fell to me. At the age of 10 I was responsible for meals and the general cleanup of the kitchen. Even though it seemed awfully early to work in the kitchen alone, I learned so much so everything has a silver lining. Even though times were hard and seemed unfair, good has come out of it. I have learned and enjoyed working in the kitchen my whole life. I've found a great deal of fulfillment there. I also remember coming home from school and finding her tucked in bed.

She so wanted to hear how our day went and was very interested but getting up to interact with us was just too much for her. I do think the hardest thing was the mood swings.

Often times when we would come home from being out, you would wonder in the back of your mind what was behind the door? Was it a mother who was happy to see you or someone who was angry because of something unforeseen? No doubt it was hard on her too, but it was downright scary sometimes for me as a little one. Like I said in the beginning, good has come out of it. Now I believe as I interact more with others, I too can sympathize with them when they deal with loved ones who are ill. We all need to do our part and use what we have experienced for the betterment of others around us!"

Love, Denise

There's a fine line between cuddling and holding someone down so they can't get away.

CHAPTER 21

WHAT DOESN'T DESTROY YOU WILL MAKE YOU STRONG!!!!

Heidi never did enjoy family gatherings. Was she the odd man out or was she like Joseph, not fitting in?

Some of the people in Heidi's family were fairly serious and she was one of them. She found her siblings a difficult lot to be a part of.

She was fortunate to marry a man with a good sense of humour. However, due to her serious nature she could be very sensitive and have difficulty laughing at times. Through the years, she has learned to laugh more and thanks to Franz, she tries to be less intense about life.

Having lost her mother at such a young tender age, Heidi found herself wanting to spend time with women who were her dear mothers' age. No doubt she was looking for that void to be filled in her life. A void that had been there since her mother died .

She remembers as a kid, she loved to spend time at her friend's house because it was special to be with their loving family. No doubt there were problems in their families too, but in Heidi's eyes their family was perfect.

When Heidi got married, she fit in well with her husband's family who loved and adored her. That was a real plus, but as time went on, Heidi wanted to see harmony in her family with her siblings.

No doubt, because of issues that had not been resolved from childhood, there was still much anger in the family.

One weekend after a dinner party, there was an argument, and as it got heated, Dianne, one of Heidi's sisters, said to Heidi, "I don't want to talk to you again except when I have to, like once a year. Only at Christmas."

Heidi was stunned! She began to share her heart with the five siblings who sat around the table.

"Over the years," Heidi began, "I've experienced rejection and I believe this is why. I know some members of the family choose to gossip and judge people and I'm not into that. No doubt this is a problem for some and perhaps feel guilty about slandering. We all make choices in life. Is there discomfort when I'm around because I care not to join in rumours and small talk? Small people talk about people, average people discuss events, and big people share ideas.

"Over the years, I've chosen at times to stay away from family because the stress of feeling shut out is too painful," bewailed Heidi as a lonely tear rolled down her cheek. "I'd rather spend time with family and friends who accept me as I am and who enjoy being together."

The weekend was horrifically painful. Her children heard and saw her pain. They warned her to stay away from people who hurt her.

The rejection Heidi felt from some of her siblings was very painful. She went home to her family who loved her dearly. She got hugs from her grandchildren.

"Mom," her son and daughter stated, "You don't need people like that in your life. Surround yourself with those who love and encourage you."

"Thanks kids, that is what I've purposed to do," Heidi answered.

Consequently, Heidi stayed away from sibling gatherings for two years. The family was stunned and begged her to come back, but as psychology states, stepping back is needed for a time in order for healing to take place.

It is much better in conflict resolution to identify the problem and together attack the problem rather than each other. People who have been abused as children often grow up wanting to control others.

"In my journey in life," Heidi reflects, "I am learning to discuss issues with my coach. These are people in my life who bring mutual respect."

Heidi adores her children and grandchildren, and she is so grateful for their love and support.

I used to be indecisive. Now I am not so sure.

CHAPTER 22

A TREASURE HUNT

As Heidi continues to be pro-active in her journey, she continues to learn through reading, etc. Heidi feels a lot of empathy for families who constantly struggle with relationships issues.

One way to get a handle on this is to start communicating. The only way to work through difficulties in relationships is to communicate. Some people are not ready to communicate and continue in their pain, meanwhile hurting others.

There are questions each family member can ask themselves. After each one answers these questions for themselves, the questions can be pooled. From those answers, the family can put together a Mission statement. A Mission statement is an agreement a family makes to help a family bond. It takes into consideration the likes and dislikes of each member, learning how to enjoy, have fun and appreciate one another through communication.

When a family has problems, they can go to their Mission statement and review it. That can bring back the respect, etc. that may be missing.

Here are some questions to help a family make up their mission statement.

What is the essential purpose of your family?
Do we want to be a family that has mutual love and respect?
Do you enjoy inviting your friends to your home?
What makes you want to come home?
Do you feel comfortable in your own home? Why or Why not?
Are there any changes you'd like to see in your family? If yes, what are they?
Are there things that embarrass you about your family?
How often are you strong enough to apologize?
How often can you forgive?
Is kindness an area we all need help in?
How well do we communicate?
Do we enjoy and appreciate each other?
How do we play and have fun?
What is synergy?
SYNERGY IS A WORKING together. It is a working together cooperatively. A family that has a deep respect for each one's varied interests and approaches is creative and fun. When there is variety and humour in a family relationship, tremendous capacity is unleashed.
If a family is truly synergistic, they will turn any challenge into a positive experience.
What is our choice? Positive or negative experience?
Like a garden-F A M I L Y-needs tender loving care. TLC

To be sure of hitting the target, shoot first and call whatever you hit the target.

CHAPTER 23

TENACITY - RESILIENCE!

Heidi needed tenacity on her winding challenging journey of life. What is tenacity? Tenacity is persisting, persevering, being steadfast, stubborn and resolute.

You may have your plans for life. Suddenly, an accident, an illness, loss of a job or the death of a loved one, knocks you off your feet. You slow down for a while. Because you are reaching for a goal, nothing will stop you from reaching your destination!

Giving up comes naturally. There is no real effort required! Ask yourself, "Am I giving up?"

"No, I am not giving up!" speaks Heidi vehemently. Heidi has worked very hard on her life's journey.

Tenacity holds fast, does not stay down when knocked down. Yes, you may be knocked off course for a time, but DO NOT RELINQUISH your plans or throw up your hands. You make adjustments and continue on.

Heidi worked very hard on her life's journey. Many relationships have been fractured because people give up! At times, marriages deteriorate to nothing. I ask you, stop and think. Ask yourself, when you were dating, did you put effort into having a good relationship? Both partners must be tenacious and put forth effort into making their relationship work. Reach for your goal, never give up!

Heidi and Franz have been married forty-five years. Was it difficult at times? Definitely yes! Did they feel like giving up? Yes, but they decided they have many, many more great memories than difficulties. They will be steadfast, and resilient.

What is RESILIENCE?

Rebounding, rapidly recovering.

HELEN KELLER overcame deafness and blindness by having a person in her life who recognized the potential in Helen. Her spiritual teacher had strength and power for her own journey. This, in turn gave her purpose and hope for Helen.

Each one of us can search for people in our lives who love us, can coach us and encourage us. This will help build resilience against helplessness.

1.Heidi's mother had resilience in life. She and Dad had a goal. They wanted a big family. They reached that goal, in having six children. Illness took Mother's life when she was only thirty-seven years of age. She left her children with a resolve to continue her tenacity and resilience!

2. Heidi had a sports injury at sixteen years of age. This left her dragging her right leg, extreme fatigue and loss of control of her right hand. At times, she fell due to balance problems. Never give up is Heidi's motto in life. There had to be an answer out there to help her with her challenges. Heidi gashed her forehead open, sprained a finger and fell into the ocean. She survived!

1. In time, Heidi learned she had Multiple Sclerosis. She learned to use a cane, then came the wheelchair. SHE DID NOT GIVE UP! She sought alternative therapy!

2. There had to be a reason for her physical challenges. She continued to look for answers.

   a. resting when her body told her to
   b. exercise

c. eating whole foods, lots of veggies and some organic meats

d. the right supplements

e. coaching encouraged her

3. Heidi's physical challenges started when she was sixteen years of age due to a sports injury. When she was sixty-two years of age, she learned how MS could be traced to a blocked vein in the neck. That made so much sense to her.

4. Right after Heidi's injury happened, her right leg started dragging and her right side went partially paralyzed.

Heidi is TENACIOUS which has resulted in RESILIENCE NEVER-GIVE-UP!

Going to church doesn't make you a Christian any more than standing in a garage makes you a car.

CHAPTER 24

HUMOUR

Thankfully, Heidi was married to a man with a great sense of humour.

Franz and Heidi loved to watch Red Skeleton on television and he was a hoot. He'd stand up on stage in his clown suit. He always had a huge impish grin on his face and would give the audience hilarious tips for a happy marriage.

He'd say – "Two times a week, my wife and I go to a nice restaurant where we have a little beverage, good food and companionship. She goes on Tuesdays and I go on Fridays!" Then Red would laugh hilariously.

"We also sleep in separate beds. Hers is in California and mine is in Texas."

Then Red Skeleton went on to say, "I take my wife everywhere...... but she keeps on finding her way back."

Franz and Heidi would have a good laugh before they decided it was bedtime.

It was great to laugh! They needed a good balance in their marriage with physical, spiritual, emotional, and mental needs. Communication-a constant challenge!

A wife needs conversation and affection from her husband.

A husband needs sexual fulfilment and to feel successful in life.

Heidi read books, she worked hard on her marriage. She learned and wanted to validate Franz. "Why was it so hard to do that at times?"

Heidi needed physical and emotional security. Her dear husband had his own issues to deal with. He owned and ran a business. He was in demand six out of seven days a week. She helped with financial and employee management. This was crucial for a successful business. At times, she did enjoy working with her husband in the business. Other times, she was so disturbed with the stress of it all.

After years of this constant juggling of finances, Heidi's body told her-I've had enough!

By this time, Heidi's eyes saw double and she knew she had to see a doctor. After many tests and probes, she was diagnosed with Multiple Sclerosis. She was not shocked-only relieved that finally she had some answers for peculiar behaviours her body kept manifesting.

Franz patiently supported Heidi when she needed extra rest and time off from the hectic business operations. He drove Heidi to the hospital for various tests the specialist needed.

They had good dependable employees who looked after details at work.

A few months after Heidi was diagnosed with the MS, she made a decision. Now that she knew what her body was dealing with, she would resign from her position at work. She knew she needed to alleviate as much stress in her life as possible. This was imperative.

Franz and Heidi travelled to California the following year. Heidi was very grateful to be released from her responsibilities at work. These two needed to get away to discuss plans for changes in the business. Little did they know that an answer was just around the corner.

Franz was not happy with Heidi's decision to step away from her position in the business. Heidi however, knew she'd done the right thing.

They were travelling to California. Their cellular telephone rang. "Hello," spoke Heidi. The voice on the other end said, "hi mom, this is Donny."

"Hi Donny, how are you?" and more pleasantries were exchanged.

"There must be a reason you called."

"Yes," he spoke, "there is. I would like to buy the business."

The conversation continued and there was their answer! Yes, their son bought the business and Heidi was elated. She totally trusted their son and knew this was the best decision. Donny was totally reliable. They trusted him implicitly and knew the business was in good hands. He'd worked in the business for seven years and knew it well. Heidi and Franz knew they could go on holidays anytime as Donny was in charge of the business. They were so grateful for that. What a relief!

Franz struggled with this decision but he didn't want to work in the business unless he could depend on Heidi. Heidi was worn out and couldn't handle the stress anymore.

When I attempted to fight fire with fire, remember that the Fire Department usually uses water.

CHAPTER 25

FAMILY SECRETS

"My poor, poor Grandpa."

It was a dismal Saturday evening. Grandma Jones sewed the last sleeve on the garment Heidi was to wear to school on Monday. How Heidi loved to caress the white stitches her grandma so patiently and lovingly stitched onto the delicate green fabric. It was a long sleeved satiny blouse which felt silky smooth.

"I wonder where Grandpa is?" questioned Grandma with alarm in her voice! "It's getting dark out there, I'd better go and see where he is. Maybe he has fallen or something."

Grandma quickly set down the new blouse and put her sweater on. Grandma knew Grandpa had been very depressed again the last while but hadn't known how to help him.

Grandma hurried out the door saying, "Heidi and Tommy, you two had better get to bed, it's getting late!"

Grandma quickly walked across the yard, through the fence and out into the field.

She called, "Henry, where are you?"

She continued to walk at a faster pace, her heart pounding as her thoughts raced!

"Oh I do hope he hasn't been foolish again," she pondered as her mind raced to the last time a year ago when she'd found him walking aimlessly by the pond soaking wet!

She'd found him with his clothes still dripping on him! As a result, he got so sick and came down with pneumonia. He almost died, but because of Grandma's loving care, he was nursed back to health. Grandma remembered that dismal time of her life! She'd thought every day for a week that he was dying.

As Grandma hurried along she kept straining her eyes out across the field to see if she could see anything. It was dark by now and she could hear the coyotes howling in the distance.

"Henry, Henry, oh where could you be?" thought Grandma. "Did you fall or are you still out here?"

Grandma's heart was racing as she was so stressed about Grandpa! Grandma knew Grandpa had been very despondent again lately. He kept losing his job and the family had to move to another farm or another town to find yet another job.

"How long would this one last?" he asked himself.

Grandpa had come from a troubling childhood. His dad had been abusive and two of his sisters had died from malnourishment.

Grandpa was delighted to marry the love of his life . She was a lovely blond with sparkling blue eyes. She was the spirited, warm-hearted daughter of his employer. This young lass joked with the farm worker every day. Catherine's job was to pack the eggs into cartons and prepare them for market.

Grandpa worked on the farm feeding the animals. There were sheep, cows and goats. Then there were white and brown chickens. The eggs from these chickens had to be gathered into big yellow baskets. Then Grandpa took the eggs into the basement of the farm home and washed each egg. These eggs were then sold to the neighbours in the community.

Dirk and Catherine-who became my grandma and grandpa-looked forward to their meeting while they worked with the eggs.

In time, the two had romance and a wedding ensued. They birthed two cuddly sweet daughters and what a delightful family they were. Dirk was extremely fond of his girls.

The pain of the past however, left him with a lot of baggage he didn't know how to cope with. His emotional baggage was like a one hundred and fifty pound load on his back which he carried day after day after day. His old thought patterns went round and round in his head every day.

They went something like this. "I can't find a job. If I find one, who knows how long it will last? I always do something stupid and quit because I feel so ashamed. What would my dad say if he saw me? He'd probably beat me over the head and call me a slob."

Poor Grandpa was in a sorry state – broken, bleeding and wounded. He didn't know how to get out of that state.

Grandpa was sitting in the field leaning his tired back against an old tree trunk.

"This is it," he said to himself. "I've struggled long enough. I can't handle this pain anymore." Grandpa slowly – oh so slowly put his hand into his pocket.

After supper, when he'd left the house, he'd stopped at the barn and picked up a handful of rat poison. "Tonight is the night," he determined within himself. "I will not have anymore pain!"

Grandma searched and searched for him. Suddenly, she heard a faint moaning in the distance. She cupped her ear. Where was this terrifying moan coming from? It sounded like Grandpa. Grandma ran toward the direction of the moan.

Then she saw him. Running ever so swiftly, she found him lying in his blood! His eyes rolled and Grandma knew this was the end. Grandma held his head in her arms and wept! With Grandma's help, he made his peace with God and died!

Besides his pain from the past – did he have a brain chemistry deficiency? Did he have a THYROID and perhaps an ADRENAL problem which can be totally debilitating?

He needed help !!

HE NEEDED HELP FOR HIS BODY, SOUL AND SPIRIT!

CHAPTER 26

THE MYSTERY OF DANCE

Over the years, Heidi noticed a delicate hormonal dance going on inside of her. It took different forms.

Depression, what's wrong with me anyway?

Weeping-why do I have the occasional outburst of weeping incessantly?

Irritability – anxiety-evil thoughts-scary!!!

Severe fatigue – debilitating – totally stressed out – resting was the only solution!!!

Falling and balance problems! Stiffness in the legs. They felt so-o-o heavy!

With life's pace – polluted air, contaminated water and questionable foods – our bodies react with fatigue and illness.

The thyroid gland is tiny, yet extremely powerful. It controls all chemical reactions of all body organs! It regulates every minute cell growth and body function as well as controlling our body temperature. The adrenal gland works closely as well.

When Heidi needs adrenal support, her mind feels anxious and her head feels upset. She is not feeling like her normal settled self. She gets irritated more quickly. She analyzes her body and mind. "What is going on?" she asks herself. "Oh yeah, I've run out of my adrenal support." After contemplating that for a few days, Heidi realized she'd better get to the health food store and get what she needed. After she replenishes her adrenal support, her mind settles down again.

When these minute cells are not getting the nutrients they need- they cannot give our bodies the energy they need. This is like the throttle in our vehicles. If the car is not getting the gas it needs, it cannot run properly.

Sometimes Heidi asks herself, "Am I ill and dying, or do I just feel that way? My energy is zip." Heidi sighs.

Life was unreasonably difficult! At times, evil thoughts would enter her mind and she would cry out to her friend who was always there to listen!! Thank God He did!!!!! It was frightening!! Heidi would have to cry out again and again – HELP! HELP ! HELP It would happen again and again. Heidi was at the end of her rope!

"Is ending my life the only answer here?" Heidi asked herself. "No, there has got to be a better answer. I will continue to search and search-there has to be a way out of this dilemma!"

"I have so much to live for," thought Heidi, "My family-I love them so."

Is low thyroid caused by a poor immune system? There is no doubt that the trauma of her mother's death and subsequently adapting to a stepmother caused much stress for Heidi. The struggles in the family of siblings added to her stress. Perhaps they were all struggling in their own way?

Heidi complained to her doctor of low energy many, many times. The blood test for thyroid returned normal and she was constantly told that tests showed no problems.

One day, Heidi walked into a naturopath's office.

In his kind, gentle manner he asked, "How are you doing?"

She responded with, "I feel like I'm barely hanging on and not sure how long I can last!"

The warm kind-hearted doctor then took her temperature. He soon left the office and returned with two containers. "I'd like you to try this thyroid and adrenal support. This works for many of our patients."

With hope for a brighter tomorrow, Heidi left the office and within the week she noticed a marked difference with her stress level.

"Wow, this is awesome, " she thought to herself. "I do feel better mentally and physically!"

In time, Heidi wanted help from the medical profession via laboratory reports and proceeded to do more research.

Through the years, a thyroid condition had been alluded to by a few doctors, but as the blood tests always showed normal, there was no reason to suspect Heidi had a thyroid problem. Over the years, several doctors identified a thyroid problem.

It was not pursued and therefore not treated. Did those doctors identify a bulge in the front of her neck and see a thyroid problem? Perhaps.

As she was one to 'never give up', Heidi found a book one day entitled Thyroid Power. She read this book fervently and oh, what morsels she found. Not only did she find answers including how to diagnose, it also had many examples and stories about individuals who suffered as Heidi did.

As Heidi researched the thyroid gland's failure to work at optimum levels, she read that there could be symptoms like:

1. suffering constant fatigue

2. suffering with depression

3. feeling hot and cold, often wearing socks to bed

4. feeling anxious, sometimes leading to panic

5. a history of thyroid problems in the family

6. having trouble with memory, feeling sluggish and trouble focusing

7. having problems with digestion resulting in feeling bloated and flatulence

8. aches and pains in muscles and joints

9. neck injuries which could have damaged the thyroid

10. feeling totally exhausted by evening and yet having trouble sleeping

Due to complications with the medical and naturopathic physicians, Heidi ran into some challenges. She wanted to know if the laboratory blood tests would prove she truly had a thyroid problem, and proceeded to find a helpful practitioner.

She found information that suggested some patients discovered that after seven doctors, they found help for their thyroid problem. Because each body is different, it is not always a black and white issue.

Finding a doctor who would work with her in this journey was another difficulty. She also learned how important it was to be pro-active.

We can empower ourselves to find some answers to our dilemma.

NEVER GIVE UP!

Heidi always found it difficult to get up in the morning and get going! She dragged herself out of bed each morning. On a good day, she'd make a list of all that she wanted to accomplish that day and before she'd completed the list, Heidi already knew she might get to number two on a list of ten. She felt fatigued just making a list!

She always had difficulty sleeping. Why was that, she asked herself. Through the years she'd buy three different products off the shelf at a pharmacy and use them on a rotation basis to help her sleep. She'd buy three different products as she did not want her body to build up a resistence to one product.

Did she have a deficiency of minerals, vitamins or amino acids?

Could the air, water and food be so toxic that it was affecting her body? It seemed her body wasn't able to function optimally. Why, why, why?

"How about exercises?" questioned Heidi. Did she need to do more? She didn't have the energy, so how could she? She learned that deep breathing was helpful several times a day.

Did she have allergies? Was there a continuous inflammation in her body? Another energy drain? Were there intestinal parasites she needed to get rid of?

Heidi eventually learned that low thyroid and adrenal problems can make any condition worse.

Is there family history of thyroid problems in the familial line? Heidi does know that an aunt of hers fainted due to a thyroid problem. Some sisters also had thyroid conditions. Yes, it was in the family.

As a child, Heidi was dizzy every morning before getting out of bed. As she sat up in bed, she'd have to sit a minute and allow the dizziness to leave before she got up. Was this indicative of a thyroid problem? Perhaps.

What comes first, depression or fatigue? Heidi believes one can cause the other!

Heidi always had cold feet. Why was that? Circulation problems caused by a low thyroid?

Heidi has always loved music. When she was a child, she taught herself to play songs on the piano written in the key of C. These songs were more straightforward to learn and she'd sit at the piano for hours and play.

Through the years, she'd occasionally hum a tune. She wondered why she hummed so seldom. Since Heidi has discovered the reasons for her weariness and continues to improve in health, she feels more like singing. Singing takes energy, and through the years, Heidi seldom had the energy to sing. What a startling conclusion! Now she loves to sing.

Heidi found a medical doctor that would work with her, and after she learned that the blood tests confirmed she had LOW THYROID, she knew she needed thyroid support. After analyzing her body and putting the information together, Heidi went to her medical doctor and asked for thyroid medication. The kind doctor agreed she had low thyroid and readily gave her a prescription. Heidi never gave up!

Now Heidis' anxiety is not there. She uses thyroid and adrenal support.

She is able to be more focused as well as not feel as mentally sluggish.

Heidi is one excited lady as this puzzle begins to fit together piece by piece.

YOU BET A CHEMICAL IMBALANCE CAN AFFECT THE BRAIN!

We lose the joy of living in the present when we worry about the future.

CHAPTER 27

HEIDI'S SPIRITUAL JOURNEY

Heidi was raised in a home where her parents spoke about faith in God. She was only six years old, but she can remember coming home from church one evening where she'd heard the preacher talk about sin. Heidi's little heart was pounding, but she was so afraid to talk about this. When the family got home, this little six year old talked about the three-letter word. S I N, what could this be? Heidi was young, but the teaching she had was indeed prevalent. She knew the difference between right and wrong. She knew what it meant to tell a lie. She knew what stealing a cookie meant.

Her little grandson, Thomas who is now fourteen years old, had that same heart throb at four years of age. One day, he spoke to his mommy about it. Mommy thought he was a little young, but when questioned, he was certain about his little life at that age. He also knew the difference between right and wrong.

As Thomas' mother explained to him, "Jesus wants to come into your heart."

Jesus, who is God's Son, died on the Cross for our sins. When we get old and die, because we've asked Jesus into our heart, we can go to heaven and live with Jesus. We will not sin anymore in heaven and we won't have any problems. We'll never have sickness or pain. We will be dancing with Jesus on streets of gold. We will laugh and sing and be happy all the time. Thomas and Zach, two of Heidi's grandsons, asked Jesus into their heart when they were four years of age.

It is awesome!! God is Heidi's strength, when times are tough, Heidi calls on Him-it's so neat!!. He is there all the time waiting for Heidi!!

When Heidi was diagnosed with Multiple Sclerosis, she'd gone to the doctor with double vision and tingling in different parts of the body. Needless to say, her general practitioner was shocked to discover what the tests showed. For Heidi, it was a relief to finally have a diagnosis. Now she knew what she had to deal with. In time, she learned to use a cane and a wheelchair because she had more difficulty walking.

It was a Sunday evening when Heidi's husband Franz and her were sitting and watching TBN-a Christian show on the television. Benny Hinn and Oral Roberts(two preachers) healing ministries were being compared. As Heidi and Franz watched people running across the platform, excited and praising God for healing, Heidi quietly thanked God for healing for the people. Heidi was still a doubting Thomas and tried to convince herself that God heals and was happy for all those individuals who were healed.

Suddenly, Heidi felt a warmth flow – ever so gently – from the bottom of her legs to the top of her legs.

She inwardly thought, "This is interesting."

Heidi softly called across the room, "Franz, do you know what I just felt? I felt a warmth flow up my legs."

Franz and Heidi got up off of their soft plush reclining chairs, hugged each other and danced around.

After a minute of that, Heidi decided to see if any changes had happened in her body. She was stunned when she was able to bend her knees and get down on the floor without any help. She got up off the floor just as easily.

When Franz saw that, he exclaimed, "That's a miracle!!!"

Two weeks before this, Heidi had tried to look into a bottom cupboard for a utensil. She had to hang onto a chair and slowly, oh so slowly, bend down while she moved her legs with the help of her hands to get her knees onto the floor. Then the getting up again was extremely wearing. Heidi was totally exhausted for the evening . This had been going on for a long time. Her legs were stiff and felt like lead. Now the stiffness was totally gone.

Heidi was ecstatic!

This truly was a very exciting part of the journey. She got a glimpse of how much better life could be, but she had more learning to do!! Lots more!.

CHAPTER 28

HEIDI'S TRAVEL FRUSTRATIONS

When Heidi was only twelve years old and in grade six, all of the class mates had to do a project on a country on this planet. Heidi and her friend Gladys teamed up. Together they decided to study Australia.

They had so much fun studying the variety of colourful birds in Australia. They also studied the many different animals like the Koala bears and the kangaroos. The girls had a lot of fun learning about the country. They worked on a booklet page by page. They had so much fun studying Australia, drawing pictures about the landscape, and the many variety of animals there were in the country. They also told about the sheep farming and the tourism business. When the girls thought they'd exhausted the study, they handed the booklet in to the teacher to be marked. The teacher was impressed and they got a good mark for the project. The girls were pleased.

After Heidi had completed the project about Australia, she'd always dreamed that one day she'd like to visit Australia.

In the year 2000, she and Franz visited Australia. They also visited Japan and New Zealand. This truly was a dream come true. Not only had Heidi been able to fulfill her life long dream, this was one of the best vacations they'd had. This time, both Heidi and Franz knew that she was dealing with Multiple Sclerosis. Now when Heidi got tired, she rested and Franz understood why and often went for a walk.

In times past, Franz sometimes got extremely irritated due to Heidi having to rest so often. The stress of the illness could cause more fatigue and frustration. Now an understanding existed which made for a more comfortable relationship.

One day on this trip, Heidi didn't have the energy to do any more walking. She spent a day in the hotel and rested. Franz went off on a tour and enjoyed watching a farmer shear his sheep. This was in New Zealand and what a wonderful time they had. The New Zealand people are a laid back kind of people and what a blissful vacation for Franz and Heidi. On this trip they visited Japan, Australia and New Zealand!

It was one of their trips to Hawaii Franz and Heidi pursued when Heidi had to go to bed due to exhaustion from travelling. Franz was not at all happy about that and let her know. "We didn't come all this way just so you could go to bed," he bitterly complained. Heidi felt badly about that but her body needed rest. There was no energy for her to do anything until she got her rest.. Admittedly, the journey of life has its challenges.

'I'm sorry,' said the clerk in the flower shop, "we don't have potted geraniums. Could you use African violets instead?" The customer replied sadly, "No it was geraniums my wife told me to water while she was gone."

CHAPTER 29

TAKE A WALK WITH ME

Heidi's battle with fatigue continued, and as long as the battle raged within her, the struggle continued. Yes, she was diagnosed with MS, but there had to be an answer somewhere! She refused to give in to the disease. Heidi would continue to learn what she could do to help her body.

Initially, Heidi fought the use of a cane, but several years later, she knew it was safer for her to use it.

Though she'd blamed her walking and falling problems on her sports injury for many years, a chiropractor was able to straighten out her spine. This treatment helped to bring healing to the body, as the oxygen could flow more freely.

Heidi had learned in her early thirties that staying off dairy products and watching her sugar intake was extremely helpful. Staying off sugar and dairy helped her beyond a doubt. Her walking improved a great deal. Eating more vegetables than fruit helped her body as there was too much sugar in the fruit for her body to cope with. One to two fruits a day suffices for Heidi.

COULD THIS HELP HEIDI TOO?

Heidi got the mercury fillings out of her teeth and had them replaced with a white composite. She called different dentists to enquire which ones were trained in how to remove the amalgams carefully. Heidi got good information and proceeded with her dentist.

The kind dentist gave her samples of composite which she took to the naturopath. The naturopath kindly tested which composite her body was best suited for. Heidi then took this information to the dentist and he performed the removal.

Did Heidi want to give up and live the rest of her life in a wheelchair if she had a choice? She'd experienced help through different avenues, so she would continue to fight with all of her might.

Yes, some days Heidi had to spend in bed, but through it all she learned that when she pushed her body too hard she suffered. Stress was a huge factor for Heidi. She had to deal with her past! She experienced a lot of therapy and got help! It was not easy to work through the pain of the past. Can it be done? Yes, it can, with tenacity and a positive attitude!

When we have damaged emotions (who doesn't have those?), we struggle a lot in life. If Heidi wants to reach her destiny, she must process her pain and tunnel through it. Our parents are not perfect and neither are our families.

It is not what happened to Heidi in her past. The question is, what is she doing with it now? Is she responding or reacting? If she continues to react, through blaming and hurting others, she will be the loser. Her health will continue to be affected.

Heidi's choice is to work with her inner self and listen to her body to continue to find answers. Meditation in the Bible helps Heidi tremendously and is huge for Heidi. Forgiveness is part of the process Heidi continues to walk through.

Getting a good night's sleep is huge for Heidi. She has learned to depend on sleeping pills to be sure she gets a good night's sleep. The medication has no side-effects the following day. Heidi is very grateful for that.

Heidi has come closer to becoming emotionally free and now she is working at helping other people. She knows there is a reason everyone goes through difficulties in life. If we take a positive attitude, we can help others in their emotional healing, which in turn helps us physically and mentally. Her eldest daughter also takes the same approach. "I can help others, because of my difficult experiences in life." What a great attitude.

Positive thoughts improve our immune system. Negative thoughts and fear-based emotions suppress our immune system. Our subconscious is like a tape recorder which plays the messages we've been programmed with since birth. If we have negative and fear-based patterns, they can eventually play out in our body.

Positive emotions are happiness, love, joy and peace. Anger can be a positive emotion, because it lets us know there is a problem we need to deal with. Negative emotions can be sadness, shame, jealousy, and rejection, and added to that can be fear and guilt. The list goes on. Ultimately, what Heidi feels deep within her determines her actions in life that she takes or does not take.

It has taken Heidi years to discover that she suffers with a thyroid and adrenal problem. She firmly believes that if she'd been aware of these challenges years ago, a lot of her depression would have been eliminated.

Let me tell you about Margaret. She had her own OBGYN practice. She suffered constantly with brain fog, dizziness and body aches. She says, "I was very moody and irritable. I'd even forget the name of my long term nurse.

I did not take my co-workers' advice to take antidepressants. I thought about many of my patients who complained of being oh so weary and fatigued. I'd been trained that adrenal fatigue is a non-issue. I followed some research and was shocked to discover how low my hormone levels were. My shortfall of cortisol and DHEA hormones triggered brain fog, exhaustion and mood swings. In Medical School, this was referred to as ridiculous, it couldn't happen. This is information physicians don't learn, because they are trained by the pharmaceutical industry.

I learned that there was action I could take to improve my health. My diet became lean and green and no caffeine, eggs, fish, poultry and little red meat, heavy on raw vegetables and a sampling of fresh fruit.

Heidi interjected, "I watch my fruit intake. I cannot handle too much sugar. I find it best for myself to eat only one to two fruits a day."

Margaret took three to four months off from her busy work schedule. During this time, she relaxed and read. She spent time with her family, truly a reprieve. Together, they went for long walks, went to the park and danced and played. After four months, Margaret was ready to return to work. She felt like a new person," finished Heidi.

When Heidi learned that a huge problem could be a chemical imbalance in the brain, she knew within her heart that she was on the right track. Her grandfather had taken his own life, so Heidi wondered if this could have had something to do with her challenges. She wondered if something in his genetics could have been passed down to her.

When the brain has a malfunction for whatever reason, the chemistry goes awry. One's thoughts can race uncontrollably when one is excited, or can become very depressed if something negative is happening in her life.

When Heidi's imbalanced chemistry was corrected with thyroid and adrenal support and her nutritional needs are met, Heidi is able to deal better with stresses.

Did her imbalance affect her marriage? Yes-emphatically yes! Her husband also has a health challenge of diabetes, which causes him to have mood swings. No doubt the health challenges have been hard on their marriage. Together, they've decided that they have many more great memories than difficult times. They'll stick with it! All of life has challenges!

CHAPTER 30

THE MISSING PUZZLE PIECE

In October of 2007, Heidi's husband alluded to a book which stated that the author found her answer to her MS. As Heidi read this book with awe, she discovered that the author was a Naturopath who'd been diagnosed with MS as a teenager. This lady also determined within herself to find an answer, and not to spend her future in a wheelchair if at all possible. This lady also discovered that the same diet Heidi pursued worked well for her.

Heidi was ecstatic. She learned that her problem could be due to a Candida Yeast infection. This blew Heidi away! In fact, within four months, she learned from three Naturopaths that this in fact could be the problem? Candidiasis? She was stunned!

Heidi learned through a lot of research that the antibiotics she'd been on for bladder and kidney infections could be part of the problem. That together with poor diet and stress killed her immune system. Antibiotics kill both the good and the bad bacteria in the gut. Hence we have problems.

Heidi immediately started on digestive enzymes and probiotics. Within a few days, her (legs felt lighter), so she knew something was happening on the inside of her body! Her legs wanted to walk stronger.

Heidi has discontinued the help of her cleaning lady because she can now vacuum. She hadn't done that in years!

Since October, when she started on this program, she's seen steady improvement. She does not use a cane anymore. She's been using a cane for some years now, so this is encouraging! Each day when Heidi exercises and follows her regimen, she gets excited because she continues to see improvement. Sometimes it's three steps forward and one step back, but oh well, hope propels her to keep going. She knows her health is so much better than she was and will continue to improve. She is so-o thankful to her creator who gave her life and walks with her every step of the way. When she falls down, He is there to pick her up.

May 2007

Heidi continues to learn via Dr. Ann's consultation over the telephone. Since May, Heidi has been more serious about the program. NO WHEAT! NO WHEAT! THAT IS DIFFICULT!

September 21st Heidi was startled when she felt like she had control of her legs like she hadn't had for years! Hallelujah! Something had happened inside her body.

Yes, it is now December and her legs get stronger as she listens to her body and follows her regimen. 1.Rest 2. Exercise 3.Diet 4.Supplements. WHAT A BATTLE!

I've noticed when I do my exercise, I can lift my legs quite easily in and out of one piece of equipment at Curves, an exercise place for women. When I started the exercises in April I had to use my arms to place my legs into the stirrup like straps. Now five to six months later I can easily lift my legs into that position. What an awesome feeling!

When I first began my exercises, my legs lifted oh so slowly. I watched the other ladies running on the spot. I thought, "Will I ever be able to do that?" My legs moved ever so slowly. By December, I was so pleased with my progress.

Heidi's mind has become more alert and focused. She still concentrates on the path in front of her when she walks. She doesn't wish to trip on a rock and throw her body off balance. Every month her body gets stronger. Her balance improves with exercise.

Heidi continues to analyze how her body is feeling with the foods she eats. She eats desserts and drinks a cup of coffee now and then. She still stays off dairy and must be careful with sugar intake. If Heidi eats wheat, it bloats her stomach and she tends to have flatulence. She tries to vary her diet and eat lots of veggies.

One night, after enjoying a potluck supper, Heidi had lots of energy. She was thrilled to be able to help with the cleanup. This was unusual and she spoke to Franz, "Did you notice I helped with the cleanup?"

"Yes," he spoke. "I was watching you."

Heidi so loves to hear this, as she is one who needs constant encouragement.

Again, Franz and Heidi took an aunt out for lunch in December. Heidi hadn't seen this lady for a year or more.

When she observed Heidi's agility in climbing in and out of the vehicle, she spoke, "What have you done to help you move so much better?"

Heidi told her and she was thrilled for her.

Would you believe that Heidi moved in December, 2009. Heidi packed and unpacked boxes like she hadn't been able to in many years. She was elated to be able to do this!

Then Heidi did a stupid thing. Franz and Heidi were together with their friends and she told her foolhardy self that she was doing so well. She gave herself permission to eat sweets and wheat and dairy to her heart's content. She ate what she wanted to. The next day, while she was moving a big chair, her energy left her. She lay down on the sofa and felt pains in her chest. After a few hours of that, Heidi's husband called the ambulance. She went to emergency and spent several hours in the hospital. Her body crashed, she was totally spent.

The good news is that, over the next few months, she discovered through blood tests that she was anaemic. Her red blood cell count had fallen constantly between May and December. With much consultation via her doctor and naturopaths, it was discovered that Heidi needed iron to build up her red blood cells. She also needed thyroid medication and B vitamins, B12 and B complex to help fight her fatigue, anaemia, muscular pains and neurological challenges.

Although it would have been better not to eat food which caused her condition to worsen, in the end she learned so much from this incident. Heidi's body needed a lot of help to build it up, and now it is getting the building blocks it so desperately needs. Yes, her red blood cells are climbing back up.

It has been a long, arduous journey for Heidi. Heidi had been pushing herself too hard, and her body crashed. She landed in the hospital. Yes, life is a learning journey.

Where would this curvy road take her next?

Who KNEW?

CHAPTER 31

NEWS FROM ITALY???????????

It was October 2009. The large colourful "new" 50" box sat in our living room. Franz and Heidi watched the 6:00 P.M. news. Suddenly, Heidi was totally focused on the broadcast blasting over the large Television screen.

Here appeared a Dr. Zamboni from Italy, a cardiac surgeon. He discovered via his wife having the MS that there could be a blockage in the neck with MS patients. The doctors in Italy had already performed a fair number of procedures in Italy. There, doctors had learned that many MS patients could be helped if the veins in the neck were unblocked. Many MS patients were being helped. Now they had a new lease on life.

His report continued as he spoke, "It seems that those with a relapsing remitting form of MS are helped the most with this procedure."

This made so much sense to Heidi. She related with what this man was saying - totally. She remembers when the injury happened. She was sixteen, and during a physical education class at school, she ran smack into the catcher. Thump! A half hour later, her leg started dragging and she felt numbness on her right side.

She believed the jar to her head or neck caused a problem? This formed a blockage in the jugular vein and blood was not able to flow to the brain and spine as it should. As a result, iron was deposited into the brain, leading to toxicity.

In fact, in her early thirties, Heidi's doctor sent her for an ECG. The report came back that she had had an injury either in the neck or at the base of the brain.

Dr. Zamboni's findings made a lot of sense to her!

Imagine

If she had a blockage, then removing the blockage, would enable the blood to circulate throughout the body so the oxygen could help heal her body. What if Heidi's brain was able to think correctly?

What if Heidi's severe fatigue lessened-what a dream!

What if her brain fog lifted totally?

She began to research this on the Internet. Yes, the procedure was being performed in India. She could go there. She discovered people were travelling to Poland, Germany, Mexico and other countries. Heidi was learning more and more about the whole process. Daily, the news was changing as people noticed a variety of changes in their bodies.

Would Canada and the U. S. join the countries in performing the angioplasty in patients who had Multiple Sclerosis?

Heidi immediately knew within herself that she was going to have this procedure done.

What could she do to help herself? She was very proactive, and knew that this was what she was going to do. There was a chance this could help her?

Many people with MS are willing to go to any length they can, to try to change their situations. They crave any improvements that might be possible inside their bodies. They yearn for more freedom all the day long.

Heidi e-mailed Dr. Ann Boroch, her Naturopath in California. She told her that she was planning to get the procedure performed for her perceived CCSVI.

What is CCSVI? A chronic cerebrospinal venous insufficiency. This means that the blood flow is constricted to the brain and spine.

Dr. Ann kindly e-mailed Heidi back and mentioned that Hubbard Foundation in San Diego was the closest place to go for the treatment.. Heidi was elated!

To be able to go to a place that close to home was energizing! Yes, Heidi could handle that! Heidi lived in Vancouver, Canada. This was not too far from home, and it was on the same continent. Yippee!

Fantastic! She was DANCING!!

CHAPTER 32

THEY WERE IN THE AIR

The airplane taxied to the end of the runway! Franz and Heidi waited and listened as the engines wound up, getting ready for take off! The steward and stewardess sat in their seats, fastened their seat belts, and waited. All passengers were buckled in their seats for safety.

This was the 10th of October, 2010.

Yes, Franz and Heidi were on their way to San Diego to have this procedure done.

Suddenly, the airplane lifted into the air. The plane climbed higher and higher up above the clouds. They soon saw blue sky.

The pilot announced, "Keep your seat belts on for safety. We are going through some turbulence!"

The stewardess began to move through the cabin. She asked each passenger what they wanted to drink. Franz and Heidi asked for some water and apple juice. They were served quickly and courteously.

After a three hour flight, the plane began descending. Soon they saw the city of San Diego in the distance. Wow, they were almost there. Excitement filled Heidi's being!

Questions Heidi had were:

1. What was this going to be like?

2. Were the doctors different here than in Canada?

3. Would her body respond positively to this treatment?

4. How long would the healing take? Would it be quick?

5. Would it be slow?

The plane landed and Heidi and Franz were soon inside the airport terminal. A kind airport employee soon brought a wheelchair. Heidi sat down in the wheelchair. The courteous attendant wheeled her through the terminal. Franz and Heidi were ushered to their destination where they picked up their rental car.

With the keys in his hand, Franz soon slipped in behind the wheel and Heidi got into the passenger side. They were off to find their hotel for the night. Franz was quick to use his GPS (global positioning system) to find their hotel that Franz had reserved.

What a nifty gadget. The GPS helped them to find their way so many times. The device saved Franz and Heidi a lot of time, as it told them which streets to turn onto to get to their destination. It also saved anxiety, as Franz did not have to depend on Heidi for directions.

They soon found their hotel and settled their luggage in the room. By this time, they were hungry. It was suppertime. A few blocks away, they discovered a Denny's restaurant. Franz parked the car, and they hurried into the building.

The hostess greeted them courteously, quickly seating them. The hostess set the menus before them.

"That chicken looks so good," spoke Heidi as she opened her menu. "I think I'll have the hamburger patty," spoke Franz.

The waitress arrived with their drinks and asked, "So what will you two have tonight?"

Heidi ordered some tasty, savoury chicken with mashed potatoes and delicious gravy.

Then Franz spoke, "I'll have a hamburger patty with mashed potatoes."

The waitress wrote the order down and then spoke, "Thank you for your order. It shouldn't be long."

The couple sat there discussing their day. "I am so happy we arrived safely." Heidi expressed. "It was an uneventful flight."

"Yes," responded Franz. "It is good to be here. I wonder what this adventure will be like?"

"I'll be happy when it's over," responded Heidi. "We've not walked this road before, so there is some trepidation."

"It will be interesting," responded Franz. "We are fearless and brave. This is something we had to do! What an opportunity."

"I agree, and I thank you so much for your support," said Heidi as she smiled at Franz. "You've always been there for me." Her blue eyes sparkled as she took his hand and caressed it.

The waitress soon approached with their delicious dinner. There were sliced cooked carrots beside the potatoes on the plate with the chicken. The service was prompt and courteous.

Franz and Heidi sat back and relaxed, eyeing their delicious looking dinners.

Franz had a little satchel and took out a pen-like object. He held it up so he could see the setting he had to turn it to. The shot was his insulin he had to take before every meal. He soon inserted the needle into his skin on his tummy. He held it there several seconds while the insulin slowly entered his body. This was done four times a day. At every meal and at bedtime.

Franz struggled with diabetes for twenty years. It was alluded to while Franz and Heidi were on a trip to Europe in 1990. Franz enjoyed his food as we all do. He suffered with swollen ankles, mood swings, and anxiety big time. However, as time went on, he was determined to control his diabetes as best he could. Desserts were his favourite and he struggled constantly with his weight. Franz really enjoyed his ice cream.

Franz and Heidi thanked God for their food, then picked up their utensils and ate heartily. They were so hungry. In a short time, the waitress returned and Franz's plate was already empty.

"Where did it go?" the waitress enquired.

"I shovelled it into my hollow leg," responded Franz as he grinned.

"You said you were hungry and now I believe you," chuckled the waitress as she picked up Franz's plate.

Heidi was always more tardy in eating her food. She savoured every bite slowly and deliberately.

After they were done eating, they paid their bill and decided to go for a little drive along the ocean. It was a lovely evening and they enjoyed the scenic drive!

The next few days Franz and Heidi spent relaxing. They scouted out a few favourite restaurants they enjoyed dining at. Dining out was a hobby they both loved to experience.

Their second night in San Diego they discovered a Mexican restaurant they especially welcomed. They knew they were not far from Mexico. They discovered there were many, many favoured Mexican restaurants in San Diego.

As they entered the restaurant, a hostess soon ushered them to a table. The spicy fragrance of the food wafted through the air. This whetted their appetites once again. A waiter hurried over and eloquently served their table with water to drink. The chips with salsa were set on their table as well. While they took pleasure in this appetizer, they revelled in the jovial Mexican music.

Heidi and Franz ordered tacos with seasoned hamburger and onions. This was topped with red and green peppers, cheese and diced tomatoes. Then green onions were sprinkled on top..

Added to this dish was the fried rice. Franz and Heidi enjoyed every morsel. It was tasty food, but these folk also knew they didn't want to eat Mexican food too often. This food seemed too rich, and they felt that one meal sufficed for a long time.

The next day, the couple went for another drive along the ocean. The ocean looked so majestic with the gorgeous mountains in the distance. Then they found it! Their favourite dining experience. It was located on the water's edge overlooking a marina with many boats and ships. What a delightful location!

While these two dined, they were mesmerized by the view. It took them back to their honeymoon experience forty-five years before. At that time they rode a ferry over to Victoria on Vancouver Island. Franz and Heidi chatted about their past forty-five years.

"Yes," chatted Heidi, "we've travelled a lot of hills and valleys in our challenging married life." "Many a couple finds that marriage can be haughty at times and humorous other times. Laugh and the world laughs with you," chuckled Franz.

They loved the expanse of water all around them The sky had a few dark and pink wisps of cloud scattered near the horizon.

"This is bliss," spoke Heidi softly.

"Yes," replied Franz. "Our life isn't over yet. Maybe the best is yet to come."
"This could be a very exciting chapter of our life," mused Heidi dreamily.

The couple ordered a tasty butternut squash soup with a very delicate flavour. This was served with a bacon and tomato sandwich which Franz and Heidi shared. For dessert, they ordered a delicious tiramisu custard with white cake and topped with whipping cream. Chocolate sauce was drizzled over the top! It was decadent.

CHAPTER 33

LIBERATION

It had been forty-seven years since Heidi enjoyed her freedom in walking. She was just sixteen years old when she'd had the trauma to her body!

Did that trauma to her body result in a blocked vein in her neck? Was this the cause of her debilitation all these years? Heidi was led to believe that this is what happened when she heard Dr. Zamboni from Italy announce the findings. Dr. Zamboni announced his findings after the treatments with some folk who had Multiple Sclerosis. Often, it was learned that the MS symptoms were relieved dramatically after a blocked vein in the neck was unblocked.

A MIRACLE!!

October 13, 2010, Heidi and Franz travelled to Del Mar, San Diego. They settled into a beautiful hotel overlooking the ocean. The large room had a King size bed with a pristine white duvet cover. Three forest green pillows accented the white cover. A small decorator orange pillow was set in the centre of the bed.

The bathroom had a double shower with new tile on the floor. There was a lovely kitchenette with everything one needed to cook a small meal. There was a small deck with a table and chairs to relax and enjoy the view of the ocean.

October 14th, Franz drove Heidi to Hubbard Foundation to have an MRI (Magnetic Resonance Imaging) scan. The imaging complete, Heidi met Devin Hubbard. The young man who was diagnosed with MS just a year before. He was the reason the Hubbard Foundation decided to add MS research to their existing research.

On October 15[th,] Franz drove Heidi to the Del Mar Vein Clinic. They'd done our scouting the day before so they knew where her procedure was taking place.

They sat down in the little office and waited. The receptionist behind the counter was friendly.

After a short wait, a nurse called, "Heidi, we are ready for you now."

Franz followed Heidi down the hall, and soon sat down to wait for the doctor. Soon, Dr. Saxon appeared and questioned Heidi.

"Have you had a lot of severe fatigue through the years?"

"Oh yes," sighed Heidi. "A lot!"

"Have you had stiffness in the legs?"

"Oh yes," continued Heidi.

"Have you had tingling in different parts of the body?"

"Yes."

"Have you had vision problems?"

Heidi responded with, "I had double vision for six weeks, and blurry vision off and on over the years."

"Do you want a stent to keep the veins open if needed?" asked Dr. Saxon.

Heidi was aware that stents in veins were controversial. She was learning that stents could work well for arteries to keep them open. Veins, Heidi was told, could collapse more easily, and a stent could then fall and float throughout the body. It could be dangerous.

"I will check your MRI and locate any problems in your body, and then we will proceed," spoke the doctor without hesitation. He then disappeared around the corner and Heidi was ushered into the procedure room.

"Please lie down on the table," kindly spoke a male nurse. "We will prep you and get you ready for the doctor."

Heidi knew that the angioplasty would be inserted into the groin area. The nurses cleaned the area with an antiseptic. At the same time, another nurse tried to get an IV needle into the arm!

"WOW!" Heidi loudly exclaimed as she felt lightning bolts pierce through her thumb.

The needle did not behave and was soon released from Heidi's wrist.

The doctor now spoke, "You're going to feel a little prick."

That was all it was, and Heidi felt more relaxed as the doctor inserted the angioplasty with the camera into the vein. With the camera inside the body, the doctor watched the screen on the wall. He pushed the balloon all the way up the veins. He watched it work its way upward, observing as the camera travelled.

It travelled past the tummy area, past the heart and into the jugular area. The balloon opened the veins as it travelled. Water was inserted into the balloon-angioplasty to enlarge the veins. It was obvious that some veins in the neck area were pinched.

Because of the blocked vein, the blood was not able to flow as it should to the brain and the spine.

As the angioplasty was pushed up past Heidi's left ear, the doctor asked, "Do you feel pain?"

"I do not have pain, but I do feel it going into my head past my left ear."

The doctor then pulled the balloon back down to the chest. He then changed directions to the right side of the neck and pushed the rod with the balloon at the end of it up past the right ear. Not long after that, he pulled all the equipment back down through the body and out of the vein in the groin.

The doctor spoke, "I got a lot of junk out of there."

Heidi immediately noticed her head felt lighter. She shook her head. Was this for real?

After the procedure, Heidi was moved from the table to a bed and transferred to another room. Here, a lovely, kind blond haired nurse attended her. For four hours, Heidi lay still while the blood was to clot. After the four hours of waiting, the doctor came by to check things out.

"Are you not behaving?" he asked. "You are being naughty."

"I know," Heidi spoke, chuckling to herself.

"We will put three stitches in and that will stop the bleeding," hastened the doctor.

Another half hour went by, and the job was complete.

Franz patiently waited all this time. Heidi met him, and together they held hands as they walked to their waiting car. Together, they went out for supper and then off to their hotel. Heidi needed to lie down and rest!

CHAPTER 34

CAN IT BE?

After the procedure, Heidi had noticed a lightness in her head. Could it be, that now that the blood was allowed to flow freely, the brain fog was lifting?

The first three days after the procedure, Heidi rested a lot. The back of her head ached, and she knew rest was best.

Fortunately, a friend had given her valid information before Franz and Heidi left their home in Abbotsford. This friend had a niece and nephew who had had this procedure done. One travelled to India and the other had flown to Mexico. These two expressed the same thoughts. They wished they'd rested more right after the procedure.

Heidi tucked this bit of information into one of the compartments in her mind. She knew when it was time, she'd put this information to good use. Because Heidi had learned through the many years of struggle with her health, it was imperative to listen to her body. If her body wasn't well, it let her know.

Here is a list of changes Heidi noticed after the procedure!

1. Her cane was not needed!! Fabulous, and her balance improved!

2. On the 4th day after the procedure, she had enough energy to take a five minute walk to the breakfast room of the hotel. Till then, Franz had brought her breakfast into the hotel room. Bless his heart.

3. Her feet were warmer and not tingly!

4. When they got home, the first morning, six days after the procedure Heidi had the energy to walk across the back lane for a cup of coffee. She hadn't done that for months, because she had had no energy.

5. She got on the stair stepper at home, and the most she'd been able to do before then was 50 steps. Now for the first time, she went on it and pumped 100 steps!!

6. She doesn't get so very tired now. This is a huge improvement.

Now, when she normally gets tired - she rests. Soon after she is ready to go again. She doesn't have to rest for hours or sometimes it was days.

7. Franz and Heidi are having guests in to dinner again. She has not been able to plan these kinds of activities for years, and now she can! Is that awesome or what?

8. Friends notice that;

    a. She looks and is more alert

    b. She looks ten years younger! Yes, Heidi likes that!

    c. She looks brighter!!

    d. She is excited about life!

    e. Her voice is louder.

9.   Her posture is much improved.

Franz and Heidi can now make plans and keep them. Heidi hasn't been able to go to the B.C. Museum for years as she didn't have the energy to walk around and look at things. Now she can do that and spend more time doing what she enjoys.

The remaining chapters in this book are thoughts and encouragement directly from Heidi. She wants to encourage those struggling through similar difficulties and give them hope for the future. As she continues her journey, she knows that her perseverance was not in vain, and that others can experience the great joy she has come to find. The one thing that she wants you to take away from this, above all other points made, is to N E V E R G I V E U P ! !

CHAPTER 35

LEARNING TO WALK?

Yes, I feel like I am learning to walk again. I tell my mind to relax. Old habits are hard to break. I ask myself, "Should my shoulders be back or somewhat forward?" I also have to tell myself to slow down. I don't need to walk quickly. I am learning to smell the flowers.

It has been six months since my procedure.

I constantly notice that little things are changing for me. I am awed at the fact that I can now actually do some shopping. When it is later in the afternoon and I feel tired, I'll go sit down. I can shop another day. I don't want to make a hurried decision, as there is no need to do that.

For years, I battled fatigue and, although learned eventually where the problem lay, I continued to fight with all of my might.

I believe that, because the blood was not able to flow to my brain and spine as it needed to, I was constantly physically and mentally challenged.

Struggles were compounded due to the loss of my insecurities as a child. The injury at sixteen years of age left me with partial paralysis and a lot of fatigue. The body is truly amazing with its resilience. The constant zeal to try again is there, I thought there must be an answer. NEVER give--------up!

I OWE A HUGE THANK YOU TO MY HUSBAND AND OUR CHILDREN AND GRANDCHILDREN!!! WHAT AN ENCOURAGEMENT THEY ARE TO ME!!!

I AM SO GRATEFUL FOR:
LAUGHTER—it happens much more easily now;
SINGING--------more energy for singing;
WANTING TO DO DISHES---------at the end of the day, some days.
MY GREAT CREATOR---------He created me;
L I F E ------through hills and valleys;
M Y MOTHER AND FATHER—they gave me life;
MY GRANDMOTHER-----------what a delight she was.

CHAPTER 36

IT HAS BEEN ONE YEAR !

I'm still challenged with my balance but it is improving.

Yesterday, I noticed I didn't need to stop at the stairs and wait before I started up the three stairs. My body felt stable and I just walked over and up the stairs. I didn't feel a need of a railing so I was extremely pleased to do that. I just discovered via the computer what exercise I need to do for my balance. I just tried it and it works! Fantastic!

I will be sixty-five years of age next year. What a thrill to have my health at this age that I haven't had in years.

The exercise I do is extremely beneficial and I deem it very important.

Rest must always come first. My body cannot be weary when I go to exercise. The other day I decided to drive to the lake and have a walk around the lake.

We live in a condo on the eighth floor. I went down the elevator and started walking to my car. My body told me, "You don't have the energy for a walk right now, you need a rest." I thought to myself, yes, I do need a rest. I turned around and walked back to the elevator and rode back up to the eighth floor. Then I entered our condo and lay down and slept. Listening to my body is so important.

I am now able to entertain. I do it carefully. I try to think about all the details and plan accordingly. If I get too tired I am still okay. I can now get away with knowing I can rest more tomorrow. It is also important to have people around that are energizing, not those who will stress me out. Stress is the worst culprit and very draining.

Yes, I've been on my own quest and found a lot of help for a cure with the Multiple Sclerosis. The journey has been long and arduous.

Is it worthwhile? Absolutely, hope is the anchor of the soul and I truly have found life to be an inspiring journey. Because of all the wonderful people I've met along my journey I am truly blessed. I've learned so much and continue to learn. What an adventure!

Words of Wisdom
"The early bird may get the worm, but the second mouse gets the cheese."

CHAPTER 37

MY DESTINY

What do I mean by my destiny? A predetermined reason to be on this earth.

I believe my destiny is to share what I have learned and am still learning in life's journey to help other people. Life is full of gems. Years of loves and losses, joys and disappointments, triumphs and failures help us figure out what is really important in life.

It is so great to live in the present, continually learning and seeking the truth in life. Experiencing life and helping others is what it's all about. This is why I was born.

Life is truly a journey when we choose to learn through challenging and sometimes hurtful experiences. The payoff comes when, through life's journey we can share stories, thereby helping others in their journey of life. Helping others work through their grief and pain is why we go through our own hurts and difficulties.

Losing my mother at five years of age, I see as the beginning of a lot of trauma in my life. My early years were tumultuous. The security I experienced the first few years of my life disappeared through the death of my mother. My father had a huge task of keeping the farm operating to make a living for our large family. That in itself was a challenge. Added to this was raising the children with love, humour and mercy.

His second wife had great difficulty handling the family. She was frazzled and nearly came apart at the seams. This dear lady lost her papa to suicide when she was only a teenager, and she was dealing with rejection from this loss.

Each one deals with rejection differently. Was this lady reacting to her childhood rejection, as she perceived her dad's suicide to be? Was she dealing with her pain by rejecting her stepchildren?

These children did not know how to deal with the death of their mother. They were looking for nurturing and loving hugs from someone who understood. The children also needed a lot of affirmation which was not forthcoming. The lady who tried to replace their mother had her own needs. Was she still reeling from her own traumatic childhood?

In days gone by, therapy was not part of one's vocabulary. Fifty years ago, if life dealt a blow, one carried on and tried to forget the past. Life has a way of teaching us through life's experiences. Memories do not disappear. We can tunnel through difficulties with positive support.

Children need much love and many words of affirmation. Does lack of this produce anger and frustration, thereby causing shame and an empty love bucket?

No doubt this can cause a lot of emotional bruises which need to be worked through in life. Failure to do so continues to whip us by our own foolish behaviour,

We can choose to understand our past, accept it and learn from it.

We can choose to be victims or we can choose to accept the fact each one of us in life goes through difficult times. It's what we do with our life that counts. Do we choose anger or denial toward our past, or do we realize that all of our experiences in life have been allowed to make us stronger people? If we choose to allow our experiences to strengthen us, we can then help others. The reality is that our attitude we take toward that life can affect our health. Our stance will help or hinder us. The choice is up to each individual.

Each individual in life needs love, affection and affirmation. We can find it through friends if we cannot find it through family.

It is hard work to bulldoze through hardships. It is a joy to learn through the journey of life and share experiences with the world. There are times I questioned whether anyone would want to hear about what I've learned. Then my inner sense takes over and says, "Oh yes, everyone can learn from others' experiences."

I am soaring higher than I ever thought!

Deeper-who ever could have imagined?

Further – Wow, what a journey!

A CHAPTER ON SUPPLEMENTS

Why do we need supplements?
We need supplements because;

1. Often the food we eat is not ripened on the vine, plants or trees

2. We are exposed to chemicals in the air, water and food

3. The food we eat is often not grown in nutrient and mineral rich soil

4. Our food is often not consumed within a few days of harvesting

5. There is much stress bombarding our body

6. We don't detoxify our bodies at least once a year

7. We need to eat a lot of fresh and raw foods

8. We often eat processed, deep fried junk food and candy

9. We don't get adequate rest in clean fresh air

10. We don't drink 8 cups of pure water daily

How IMPORTANT TO GET THE
TOXINS OUT OF THE BODY!!
I use the following supplements and they
WORK WELL FOR ME

----------------get the toxins----------------OUT-OUT-OUT OF
THE BODY!!
NOW NOW NOW NOW WITH A
P U R E L I F E C L E A N S E 15 day cleanse with no fasting
- Gentle intestinal cleanse
- Herbal detoxification www.joysinspiringmsjourney.ca
Or
COLO-VADA-PLUS

Cleanses waste out of the colon

Get the damaging toxins out of the body

Could help to eliminate parasites www.joysinspiringmsjourney.ca

DIGESTION FORMULA - plant enzymes for complete digestion
- Pro-biotics for healthy immunity
When I started on the DIGESTION FORMULA – I was BLOWN
AWAY as in a few
days I noticed my legs wanted to walk. Something was happening
on the inside of my body. I was getting the nutrients my body craved
and needed. I needed enzymes for
digestion. I was amazed www.joysinspiringmsjourney.ca

I like to take liver support as the liver is the biggest organ in the
body to absorb the many toxins and flush the body. ARTICHOKE
LIVER CLEANSE
found at www.joysinspiringmsjourney.ca

24/SEVEN My favourite multi-vitamin. Supports overall health with vitamins
and minerals plus whole foods, antioxidants, herbs and heart healthy nutrients.
www.joysinspiringmsjourney.ca

I.Q. DHA supports brain health
Helps the nervous system
Assists brain and eye function
A vegetarian source of the critical OMEGA 3 ESSENTIAL FATTY ACID.
www.joysinspiringmsjourney.ca

renew replenish rejuvenate
A formulation with Vit. D which supplies nutrition to bone marrow, which in turn helps production of healthy new adult stem cells. We need these as our body deteriorates with age. www.joysinspiringmsjourney.ca

MYNAX by Koehler alleviates my pain. A fantastic supplement in which
The combination of Magnesium EAP 105 mg 26 percent
Calcium EAP 66 mg 7 percent
Potassium 288 mg 8 percent
This takes care of all my muscle pains in my back, legs and arms!
GREAT stuff
Check it out online.

HEIDI'S FOOD GUIDELINES RECIPES

First thing in the morning 2 cups detox tea

Breakfast

1. eggs can be in the form of an omelette made with onions, celery, zucchini, avocado, and/or chicken OR

2. Oatmeal Porridge with flax, nuts and raisins Served with coconut milk or soya or rice milk.

Lunch

1. Best Burgers served with yam fries Fruit smoothie made with coconut milk and two Fruits like pineapple and strawberries OR

2. Pasta Italiana with a green salad

3. baked fish with a large fresh green salad

Supper

1. Hamburger Soup with rice flour bread OR

2. Haystacks (delicious)

Snacks for am or pm a handful of almonds OR
an apple, OR
celery sticks with almond butter. OR
carrot sticks

RECIPES FOR
Best Burgers-no meat Haystacks, Pasta Italiana, Hamburger Soup

Best Burgers ¼ c.	Chopped walnuts
1c. Water	½ tsp. salt
1 onion chopped	¼ sage
3 Tbsp. Liquid Aminos	1/8 tsp. marjoram
1clove minced garlic	1/8 tsp. thyme
	½ cup rolled oats

Bring first column of ingredients to a boil. Stir in remaining ingredients and let Stand for 10 minutes. Drop by ¼ C scoop onto a sprayed cookie sheet. Flatten and Bake at 350 F for 25 minutes, then turn and bake an additional 15 minutes.
Can also be cooked in a skillet based in olive oil.

Hamburger Soup

Sauté a large onion in olive oil	salt and pepper to taste
Sauté 1 lb. Lean hamburger meat	add 2 beef bullion
Add 9 cups water	add 3 T. Liquid Aminos
Add one cup rice	add one can green beans or
Add one cup sliced carrots	one can kidney beans
Add one cup diced celery	add one can tomato sauce

Cook for one hour and serve.

Pasta Italiana

½ lb sesame macaroni or rice   1 clove minced garlic

2 – 16 oz cans tomatoes   1 bay leaf

2- 15 oz. cans red
kidney beans, drained   1 tsp onion powder

1 can tomato sauce   1 tsp chopped parsley

½ tsp oregano   1 tsp salt

    ½ tsp sweet basil

Cook macaroni or brown rice as directed on package. Cook the remaining ingredients
And simmer for 20 minutes. Pour over rice or macaroni and serve. May also be baked
As a casserole.

Haystacks

Oven baked corn chips   chopped olives

Seasoned beans   chopped green onions

Shredded lettuce   salsa sauce

Diced tomato   guacamole

Finely diced onion

Place corn chips on plates. Then place remaining ingredients (in order) given on top of chips.

MY THANKS TO

SELF MATTERS DR. PHIL SAYS CREATING YOUR LIFE FROM THE INSIDE OUT

HEALING MS Dr. Ann Boroch

EMOTIONALLY FREE Dr. Grant Mullen M. D.

THE CANDIDA CURE yeast, fungus and your health by Dr Ann Boroch

HELP YOURSELF HEALTH CARE Dr. Albert Zehr

FACING YOUR GIANTS Max Lucado

SELF MATTERS by Dr. PHIL McGraw

THYROID POWER by Dr. Richard L. Shames M.D. and Karilee Shames R.N. PH.D

DARING TO BE YOURSELF by Alexander Stoddard

THE SEVEN HABITS OF HIGHLY SUCCESSFUL FAMILIES BY Stephen Covey

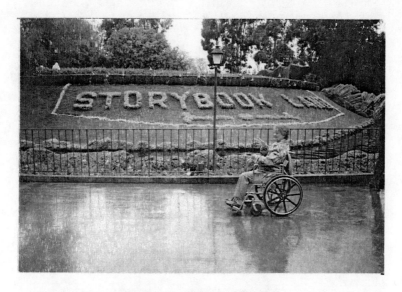

Heidi in wheel chair 1995

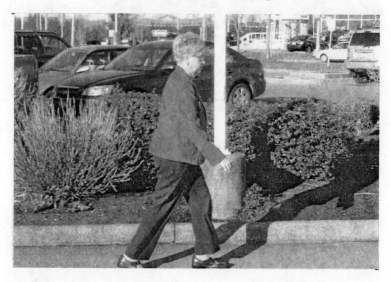

Heidi walking 2012-02-17 Thank God for A MIRACLE !

Index

Q

QUIET TIME 74

R

REJECTION 34, 87, 119, 146
RELATIONSHIPS 90, 93
  Communicating 90
  Continue in their pain 90
  Hurting others 90, 118
  Misunderstandings 77
REMOVE TOXINS 60
  Enema 58

S

Sensitivity to criticism 73
SPORTS INJURY VII, 55, 72, 94, 95, 117
STRESS 20, 65, 73, 87, 98, 99, 105, 115, 121, 143, 149
  Severe fatigue 51, 58, 66, 126, 134
SUGAR IX, 55, 57, 66, 117, 120, 123
SUPPLEMENTS 65, 95, 149, 150

T

TENACITY 15, 93, 94, 118
  Reaching for a goal 93
THYROID 103, 108, 155
  digestion 106, 150
  Feeling hot and cold 106
  Low thyroid 105, 108
TONGUE 3, 29, 56, 64
TRANSVERSE MYELITUS 8
  Virus that attacked spine 8

W

WHEAT 122
WHEELCHAIR 10, 11, 66, 67, 94, 112, 118, 121, 129
Works with thyroid 104, 105, 106, 107, 108, 119, 120, 124

CPSIA information can be obtained at www.ICGtesting.com
Printed in the USA
LVOW060802160912

298891LV00001B/11/P